MANAGING Y

HEALTH & WELLNESS

About the Author

Diane L. Cramer, M.S. (New York) is a consulting astrologer, lecturer, and teacher in all aspects of astrology who specializes in medical astrology and nutrition. She lectures for two national astrological organizations—the NCGR and the AFA. This is her third book.

To Write to the Author

If you wish to contact the author or would like more information about this book, please write to the author in care of Llewellyn Worldwide and we will forward your request. Both the author and publisher appreciate hearing from you and learning of your enjoyment of this book and how it has helped you. Llewellyn Worldwide cannot guarantee that every letter written to the author can be answered, but all will be forwarded. Please write to:

Diane L. Cramer, M.S.
℅ Llewellyn Worldwide
2143 Wooddale Drive, Dept. 0-7387-0849-6
Woodbury, MN 55125-2989, U.S.A.
Please enclose a self-addressed stamped envelope for reply,
or $1.00 to cover costs. If outside U.S.A., enclose
international postal reply coupon.

Many of Llewellyn's authors have websites with additional information and resources. For more information, please visit our website at www.llewellyn.com.

MANAGING YOUR
Health
& Wellness

A Guide to Holistic Health

Diane L. Cramer, M.S.

Llewellyn Publications
Woodbury, Minnesota, U.S.A.

First Edition
First Printing, 2006

Book design by Donna Burch
Cover design by Kevin R. Brown
Edited by Andrea Neff

Chart wheels were produced by the Kepler program by permission of Cosmic Patterns Software, Inc. (www.AstroSoftware.com)

Disclaimer: The purpose of this book is to provide educational information for the general public concerning herbal remedies that have been used for many centuries. In offering information, the author and publisher assume no responsibility for self-diagnosis based on these studies or traditional uses of herbs in the past. Although you have a constitutional right to diagnose and prescribe herbal therapies for yourself, it is advised that you consult a health care practitioner to make the most informed decisions. In particular, the herb comfrey is best used externally as an ointment or as tincture drops in water made into a compress. Do not ingest, as some studies suggest that comfrey is carcinogenic in large doses.

Llewellyn is a registered trademark of Llewellyn Worldwide, Ltd.

Library of Congress Cataloging-in-Publication Data
(Pending)
ISBN-13: 978-0-7387-0849-2
ISBN-10: 0-7387-0849-6

Llewellyn Publications
A Division of Llewellyn Worldwide, Ltd.
2143 Woodale Drive, Dept. 0-7387-0849-6
Woodbury, MN 55125-2989, U.S.A.
www.llewellyn.com

Printed in the United States of America

Other Books in the Astrology Made Easy Series

Contents

Charts

Acknowledgments

The author wishes to thank and acknowledge Kris Brandt Riske for paving the way for this book to be written, and also Stephanie Jean Clement, Ph.D., whose help was invaluable for writing this book. Stephanie never tired of answering my endless questions and was always available to guide me. I also wish to thank my editor, Andrea Neff, for her insightful comments and queries. Because of her helpful suggestions and fine editing, the book is clearer and more understandable to both the layperson and the astrology student.

Disclaimer

The information contained in this book is based on the use of medical astrology going back hundreds of years. It is informative insofar that according to ancient tradition, the planets and the signs of the zodiac are said to be associated with parts of the body and help describe the body's proneness and reaction to disease. This ancient information is presented in a modern and easy-to-use format to help the reader gain a better understanding of their physical body. However, the information gleaned from this book should in no way be used as a substitute for advice from a doctor or licensed health professional. The natal birth chart cannot and should not be used to diagnose disease. It is simply a tool to help you learn more about your body. Only a medical doctor can diagnose disease. Once the reader has determined what they perceive to be a bodily weakness or proneness to a specific disease state, they should consult a licensed medical professional for help. The publisher is not responsible for the misuse of the information contained in this book, which is offered solely as one of many tools available for improving one's health.

It should also be mentioned that various alternative health techniques as well as information on different health disorders are mentioned in this book. There will always be controversy over the causes and cures for various diseases as well as controversy over nutritional causes and remedies for health disorders. The author has mentioned the most commonly used alternative techniques and publicized information on the causes and cures for different health disorders and has depended on the medical expertise of the authors listed in the bibliography at the end of the book.

1
How a Wellness Report Can Help You Achieve and Maintain Better Health

A personal wellness report will enable you to pinpoint the weak areas of your body as well as help you determine your proneness to specific disease states based on your birth chart. The CD-ROM that is included with this book contains a calculation program that enables you to print out your birth chart in a user-friendly style that is easy to understand. Your printout will include the sign and house positions of the planets in your chart. The symbols for the signs and planets are listed. You will also be able to print out and read a personal health report that will interpret your chart in terms of medical astrology. You will be given the meanings of the signs and house positions of your planets and an interpretation of your Ascendant. Because your birth chart is used, you will be able to gather information that is tailored to a personal health interpretation.

This is the beginning of your journey to better health in that you immediately have a simple but effective way to begin improving your overall health. Astrological and medical terms will be explained throughout the book and will also be included in the glossary at the end of the book. Nutritional guidelines and techniques will also be given throughout the book as well as in appendix A.

With the help of this book, you will be able to start evaluating your bodily strengths and weaknesses. Once you determine the weak areas of your body, you can take measures to build them up. You may begin a new health regimen that includes dietary changes and lifestyle changes or choose to work with a health practitioner who meets your personal needs. You can refer to appendix A for information on how to nourish weak areas of the body and learn healing methods for some common diseases. Sample chart interpretations are provided in appendix C.

What Is Medical Astrology?

Your report utilizes the basics of medical astrology—one of the earliest forms of astrology. Medical astrology offers you a time-tested method to recognize and improve deficiencies in your body. It is the branch of astrology that deals with the planetary causes of disease. It has its origins in ancient astrology and was used by Hippocrates (b. 460 BC) and by most doctors until the seventeenth century. Medical astrology associates the different parts of the body and the illnesses connected with them with the signs of the zodiac and their associated planets. There is also a correspondence between the planets and disease in that specific planetary combinations can point to proneness to a specific disease state. As you read chapter 2, "The Signs in Medical Astrology," and chapter 3, "The Planets in Medical Astrology," you will begin to understand the correspondences between the planets, the signs, and health. You will see why medical astrology can be an important adjunct to traditional medicine.

What Medical Astrology Can and Cannot Do

Medical astrology can help you eliminate improbabilities in the chart and hone in on major themes in much the same way as natal astrology. However, medical astrology is more complicated than natal astrology. First of all, you need to be a competent medical astrologer to fully interpret a natal chart. Second, by law you cannot diagnose illness unless you are also a medical doctor. And, there are too many variables in a chart for it to be used for diagnosis. But medical astrology can help you eliminate implausibilities in your chart and focus on the vulnerable parts of your body. It also shows your strengths and the ways in which you respond to disease.

2
The Signs in Medical Astrology

The signs of the zodiac correspond to the anatomical locations in the body of tissues and organs. Along with the planets, the signs can also describe the physiology (body processes) of an organ or tissue. In many cases there are similarities between a sign in the zodiac and the planet it is associated with. For example, Libra refers to the anatomical location of the kidneys, and Venus, which is associated with the sign Libra, can describe kidney action. Therefore, kidney function in the body can be related to both the sign Libra and the planet associated with it, which is Venus. In another example, Sagittarius describes the anatomical location of the liver in the body, and Jupiter, the planet associated with Sagittarius, can describe liver function in the body.

As you learn more about medical astrology, you will discover that there is a relationship between the planets and the signs in determining proneness to specific disease states and bodily weaknesses. You will also learn that astrologers associate the planets with a sign or signs. This is called *rulership*, and in the above example of the association between Venus and Libra, an astrologer would say that the sign Libra is ruled by the planet Venus; or, taking the other example, that the sign Sagittarius is ruled by the planet Jupiter.

The planets and the signs can both have attributes that describe similar actions, such as heat and inflammation for both the planet Mars and the sign Aries. The action of a planet is influenced by the sign it tenants while at the same time influencing the sign itself. To illustrate, suppose you have Mars in Cancer in a chart. The action of the planet, Mars, influences the sign, Cancer, in that one could have an acid stomach or be prone to stomach upset when upset or angry. This is because the sign Cancer is the general ruler of the stomach and Mars is a planet promoting acidity as well as being the planet of anger and aggression. But the sign in turn affects the planet's ability to act. Mars loses some of its ability to act when in the sign of Cancer. Any beginning astrology book will state that Mars in Cancer is in its "fall" and is therefore not able to act up to par.

The list that follows gives the general associations of each sign of the zodiac and each sign's actions and reactions to disease. Included are the most recognizable parts of the body for the layperson. Since signs and planets can be involved in more than one function or location in the body and since a function of a sign can sometimes be seen in its opposite sign, which is called its *polarity*, the reader may notice some overlapping. The functions of tissues and organs in the body can be very complex and are not limited to one planet or sign.

Aries

The sign of Aries can be infectious in nature and responds with heat and inflammation. It is an energetic and impulsive sign, with a tendency to waste energy. It is involved with feverish complaints. It is associated with the head and brain, skull and face, outer ears, eyeballs, upper jaw, adrenal medulla, and pituitary gland. Aries is also linked with renal function due to its polarity with its opposite sign, Libra.

Taurus

Taurus is a sign of stability, support, and endurance. It rules the senses. It is a sign of aggregation, which can lead to tumor formation or cysts. The lower jaw and middle ears are ruled by Taurus, as are the thyroid gland and thymus gland. Taurus is also associated with the neck, throat, tonsils, adenoids, palate, vocal cords, larynx, and pharynx.

Gemini

Gemini is a sign of dispersal and flexibility, and is associated with linkages and connections in the body. It rules the tubes of the body. It is a communicator and a sign of locomotion. It rules the lungs and the process of inhalation as well as the central nervous system, arms, shoulders, hands, tongue, trachea, bronchi, Eustachian tubes of the ears, ureter, and fallopian tubes. Capillaries and collagen are also ruled by Gemini.

Cancer

Cancer is a sign that protects and nurtures. It is associated with all containers and coverings in the body. It is a moist sign and rules mucous membranes and bodily fluids. It rules the breasts, rib cage, sternum, thoracic cavity, stomach, womb, pleura of the lungs, endocardium, and pericardium. It also rules both the eye sockets and the cornea of the eye as well as the sinus cavities. Cancer is also involved in gastric digestion.

Leo

Leo is a fire sign, with much energy and vitality. It is vivifying and centralizing. In illness it expresses itself as fever and inflammation. Leo rules the muscular portion of the heart, the spine, and the middle back. It is associated with the pulmonary and coronary arteries.

Virgo

Virgo is a sign of analysis, assimilation, and discrimination. It is involved in the processes of splitting and separating in the body. It rules the small intestines, pancreas, duodenum, enzyme action of the liver, and peristalsis of the bowel. It may be involved in wheat allergies.

Libra

Libra is a sign of balance and adjustment. It adjusts and regulates in its role of keeping the body balanced. It is associated with the processes of filtration and distillation. It has rulership over the kidneys, the lower back, and the skin as it relates cosmetically. It refers to the lumbar region of the spine. It is involved in the acid/alkaline balance of the body. Like its opposite sign, Aries, Libra is involved with adrenal action.

Scorpio

Scorpio is a sign of transformation and elimination. It has great strength and endurance. It is involved in the procreative processes of the body as well as excretion. It rules the colon, bladder, ovaries, vagina, prostate gland, urethra, cecum (the first part of the large intestine), and all bodily outlets. Its nature is to throw off, eject, and eliminate.

Sagittarius

Sagittarius is a sign of locomotion and transference. It rules the exhalation process of the lungs as well as the hips, thighs, and liver. It rules the sacral region of the spine, the femur, and the sciatic nerve. It is involved in the distribution of body fat. It also rules the saphenous vein.

Capricorn

Capricorn is a sign of structure and limitation. It inhibits and obstructs and tends toward crystallization, but it is also a sign of management. Capricorn rules the skin in its role as a protector and is involved in serious skin diseases. It rules the knees, joints, hair, bones, teeth, and nails. It rules the skeleton of the body and the minerals in the body.

Aquarius

Aquarius is associated with the circulation and oxygenation of the blood. It is also associated with rare illnesses and nervous disorders. It is involved with blood poisoning and incomplete oxygenation in the body. Aquarius rules the electrolytes in the body as well as the lower legs and ankles, the valves of the heart, and the retina of the eye. It is involved in the cooperation of bodily processes.

Pisces

Pisces relates to unusual diseases, diseases that are hard to diagnose, and the misdiagnosis of disease. It rules the lymphatic system of the body, the feet, and the toes. The nature of Pisces is to soften and relax, resulting in a lack of tone. This sign has the ability to break down barriers. It is involved in the production of phlegm and mucus. It rules alcohol, drugs, and poisons. Its effects can also be psychic or mental in the case of hallucinations or obsessions.

3
The Planets in Medical Astrology

The planets in medical astrology help determine one's proneness to specific disease states, one's endurance and resistance to disease, one's nutritional needs, and much more. They are used to describe the physiology of the organs and tissues in the body. They can be interpreted by sign position or house position, or in combination with other planets. A combination of planets along with other indications such as house and sign emphases in the birth chart can describe an astrological signature that is specific to a certain disease state. This is referred to as an astrological disease significator. For example, if, when examining a natal chart, there were several stressful aspects to the Sun along with an emphasis of planets in the fifth and eleventh houses and an inclusion of the signs in the fixed mode (the signs Taurus, Scorpio, Leo, and Aquarius)—especially Leo and Aquarius and other indications such as a stressful aspect between Jupiter and Saturn—a medical astrologer might determine that there is a weakness in the heart and circulatory system.

In analyzing planetary combinations, just as in natal astrology (the study of the birth chart in terms of character and personality), rarely does one combination of planets indicate a specific trend. The medical astrologer learns to look for repetitive patterns in the chart before coming to any conclusion.

The following describes the basic nature of each planet in terms of medical astrology but does not take into account sign position, house position, or aspects between the planets, which are needed to make a proper judgment. The information is provided to help the reader understand the basic nature of each planet in terms of its action and re-action to disease. The planets have more than one function in medical astrology and are not the sole causative factor of a health disorder, as one must also take into account hereditary factors and lifestyle. This chapter will emphasize the basic nature of the planets with respect to health. See chapter 4 for a description of the planets in the signs. See chapter 5 for a description of the planets in aspect to each other. See chapter 6 for a description of the meanings of the planets in the houses.

Sun

The Sun is not a planet but a luminary, and its sign position in the zodiac and planetary aspects provide much information for chart interpretation. It is associated with the basic vitality of the cells. When the Sun is a causative factor in illness, you can expect an in-fectious or inflammatory response. You may be burning off toxins through a fever or in-fection. If your Sun receives several stressful aspects, it can indicate vitality problems or an uneven vitality. This can manifest as both low physical energy or low ego energy, re-sulting in an inability to stand up for yourself or low self-esteem. A highly stressed Sun can also point to a heart disorder or to back and spinal problems. The Sun is also asso-ciated with eye problems. The Sun rules the right eye in a male and the left eye in a fe-male. Disorders associated with the Sun tend to be acute.

Moon

The Moon, which is also a luminary, is associated with bodily rhythms, functional disor-ders, and disturbances in bodily cycles. It rules the daily rhythms of the body. It is associ-ated with fluid balance, swellings, and water retention in the body. A strong lunar influ-ence in the chart can result in allergies. This is especially true if the Moon is in one of the angular houses in the chart (house one, four, seven, or ten). The secretions of the body, as well as fluids such as lymph and serum, are associated with the Moon. The Moon is in-volved with mucus formation and catarrh. Since the Moon rules one's emotions, it is asso-ciated with psychological problems, emotional instability, and psychosomatic complaints. The Moon also rules the female menstrual cycle and any disturbances in that cycle. It is also associated with pregnancy. The Moon rules the right eye of a female and the left eye of a male.

Mercury

Mercury has rulership over the respiratory and nervous systems. It is a regulatory planet and is involved in many bodily functions. It is associated with disorders such as pneumonia and bronchitis, neuritis and neuralgia. As the planet of communication, in its role as message carrier, it is associated with the hormones in the body. If Mercury receives several stressful aspects, it can indicate a proneness to a hormonal imbalance in the body. Mercury is also the general ruler of mental and learning processes and the organs of speech and hearing. It is prominent in speech disorders such as stuttering or learning problems such as dyslexia. Mercury is also important in determining one's mental health and would be a factor in disturbances of mental health. In terms of movement and agility, it also rules the arms, hands, and fingers.

Venus

Venus is associated with the sensory system of the body. It rules the kidneys and their role in regulating the balance of the body. Kidney function or dysfunction is ruled by Venus. This planet has rulership over sugar and is associated with diseases such as diabetes and hypoglycemia. Venus also rules the veins and thus the venous circulation of the body. Phlebitis and varicose veins are Venus-ruled conditions. Venus rules the sensory organs and their ability to function. It rules the sign Libra, which has to do with the skin, and is therefore associated with benign skin growths or minor skin irritations. One's personal taste in food is associated with the placement of Venus in the chart. Venus is also a factor in body tone.

Mars

Mars refers to an overworked part of the body. Its location in the body by sign receives more heat, infection, or inflammation than other parts of the body. Mars is a fighter, and a Martian response in the body can be expressed as a high fever, infection, inflammation, or irritation. Mars is associated with aches and pains in the body and with the pain that is the result of an accident or surgery. As the ruler of accidents and operations, its sign position is vulnerable to a surgical procedure or injury. For example, Mars in Aries is susceptible to accidents to the head, Mars in Gemini is susceptible to breaking an arm or wrist, and Mars in Cancer is susceptible to abdominal surgery. The action of Mars is eruptive. Mars rules the red blood corpuscles and is involved in blood diseases such as anemia. It also has rulership over the iron level in the blood. It rules acids and acid conditions in the body. With Mars, illness can be sudden and acute. This planet also has rulership over burns, bruising, ulcers, hemorrhages, flare-ups, and muscular disorders. It is associated on a psychological level with anger and aggression. Mars is also a sexual planet and therefore describes one's sexual attitude and/or sexual dysfunction as well as one's potential to contract a sexually transmitted disease.

Jupiter

The nature of Jupiter is to expand and enlarge. Jupiter is the largest planet in our solar system; therefore, the rulership of the sign placement of Jupiter can sometimes point to a part of the body that is considered larger than normal. Jupiter is associated with fat assimilation in the body and with the arterial blood circulation of the body. Excess cholesterol in the body can be related to Jupiter. The distribution of body fat is associated with this planet. Persons with Jupiter strongly placed in the chart can have a tendency toward weight gain. A planet in an angular house (house one, four, seven, or ten) is considered a strong placement. Jupiter refers to diseases caused by excess, and is also associated with engorgement and swelling. Jupiter has to do with "too much," such as eating, drinking, or immoderation in general. It is associated with gout. Jupiter also has a protective function and can help in the preservation of health. It can sometimes be seen as a guardian angel.

Saturn

Saturn has the function of protecting the body in its rulership of the bones and skin. However, as the planet of limitation, it can indicate vitality problems and chronic disease. The sign it tenants is considered to be the weakest point in the body, due to a weakened blood supply. This point or organ can be underdeveloped in some way. It is a part of the body that needs to be guarded and nourished. Where Mars is acidic, Saturn is alkaline. Saturn is involved with hardening, retention, crystallization, calcification, obstruction, underactivity, and failure. Stiffness in the body is Saturn-ruled, as is a blood clot. Saturn is involved with malignancy, atrophy, and chronic weakness. Food disorders such as malnutrition are associated with Saturn. Deafness and dental problems are Saturn afflictions. Serious skin diseases such as psoriasis, eczema, and skin cancer are also associated with Saturn.

Uranus

Uranus can indicate sudden and unusual illnesses. Uranus has general rulership over the circulatory system and circulatory disorders and is also involved with heart palpitations and arrhythmia. It rules the valves of the heart. It is associated with spastic conditions, cramps, convulsions, ruptures, incoordination, seizures, twitching, and diseases such as epilepsy and Parkinson's disease. Uranus rules shock, so it would be involved in accidents with electricity or lightning or in the use of shock therapy. Stress-related illnesses are also ruled by Uranus. Conditions from restlessness to a nervous breakdown are Uranus-ruled.

Neptune

Neptune is considered a difficult planet in medical astrology, as its nature is to hide, deceive, and disguise. It can be diffusive and weakening. There can be misdiagnosis, a hidden illness, or an inability to diagnose a medical problem when Neptune is involved. Neptune is associated with drugs and alcohol and is present under conditions of alcohol or drug addiction or drug overdose. Neptune strongly placed in the chart can indicate someone who is drug-sensitive or who is prone to allergies. As mentioned previously, a strongly placed planet is usually a planet in an angular house (house one, four, seven, or ten). Neptune has rulership over the immune system and is also involved in malignancy and mastitis. Neptune rules poisons and pollutants. The sign relating to the part of the body it tenants can be flabby, with a lack of tone, and needs to be nourished and built up. Neptune is involved with delusions and hallucinations or anything that distorts reality. It rules coma and the unconscious and disorders that begin in the subconscious. Like Pluto, it rules bacteria and viruses.

Pluto

Pluto is the planet of transformation. It is associated with cellular division and hereditary diseases and is involved with birth defects and genetic disorders. It has general rulership over the endocrine system. It is associated with massive infection, inflammation, abscess, malformation, and malignancy. It is involved in the transformation of the body, for better or worse. Transplants, as well as surgical operations and amputations, are ruled by Pluto. A drastic health situation or an abnormal growth is Pluto-ruled. Pluto also rules bacteria, viruses, and parasites. It can be eruptive or purging in nature.

4
The Planets in the Signs

Each planet in your chart and its sign placement can give you information about your health. As described in chapter 2, each sign of the zodiac is associated with particular parts of the body and their actions or reactions to disease. And as described in chapter 3, each planet in your chart is associated with a particular type of action, which in turn influences and is influenced by the sign it occupies. The information that follows is concerned with the planets in the signs.

Sign placement is used along with the planetary aspects to find a particular theme in a chart. Sign placements, which are associated with the anatomical locations in the body, can help the medical astrologer pinpoint potential trouble spots in the body. One should also note the connection between a planet in the chart and the sign it is associated with, or rules. For example, when reading the descriptions of Venus in the signs, one will note the relaxing effect of Venus on an organ as well as its relationship to kidney action and to the throat. That is because Venus rules Libra, the anatomical location of the kidneys, and it also rules Taurus, the anatomical location of the throat.

For information purposes, the reader can refer to the following list of standard acceptable planetary rulerships:

The Sun rules Leo.

The Moon rules Cancer.

Mercury rules Gemini and Virgo.

Venus rules Taurus and Libra.

Mars rules Aries and ruled Scorpio before the discovery of Pluto.

Jupiter rules Sagittarius and ruled Pisces before the discovery of Neptune.

Saturn rules Capricorn and ruled Aquarius before the discovery of Uranus.

Uranus rules Aquarius.

Neptune rules Pisces.

Pluto rules Scorpio.

You may also find that a bodily weakness exists in one of the four signs of a particular mode or modality. In other words, you may have Saturn in Taurus (a fixed sign) but can also experience attributes of the other signs of the fixed mode or modality—Scorpio, Leo, and Aquarius. As you will learn in chapter 9, the three modes are the cardinal signs: Aries, Libra, Cancer, and Capricorn; the fixed signs: Taurus, Scorpio, Leo, and Aquarius; and the mutable signs: Gemini, Sagittarius, Virgo, and Pisces.

As stated, the following information illustrates vulnerable areas of the body based on the planet and the sign. The information is given so that you can begin to nourish these weak areas. It should also be noted that one indication in a chart is not enough to assume a proneness to a potential disease. It takes several astrological significators—including planetary aspects, planets in signs and houses, and other indications such as elements and modes—before one can make an assumption of a potential disease.

The reader will note that various remedies are mentioned to help prevent or treat various disorders. It goes without saying that if you suspect you have a serious disorder such as heart disease or are suffering from symptoms from an undiagnosed problem, only a qualified health professional can help you. Any of the following treatments that are mentioned should be discussed with your doctor.

The Sun in the Signs

Each Sun sign is associated with vulnerable areas of the body in accordance with the parts of the body associated with, or ruled by, that sign. These can be considered hot spots in the body, which could describe a weakness in these parts of the body or lead to a potential disease when stressed. The information that follows describes one type of characteristic—a planet in a sign—and can be modified for better or worse by other factors in the chart.

The Sun provides information on your physical vitality, metabolism, resistance to disease, and ego development. Solar responses tend to be feverish, inflammatory, and infectious and affect one's vitality. The sign position of your Sun provides much information on your strengths and weaknesses.

Sun in Aries

This is a sign of physical robustness, vitality, and vigor. You are happiest when on the go and involved in activities that use your boundless physical energy. You are rarely tired and can work for long periods of time without a break. You can be headstrong and aggressive, with a tendency to be impatient and hasty. You like to live life in the fast lane, and your impulsiveness and impatience can sometimes lead to falls, cuts, or bruising. This can be prevented by wearing protective gear when involved in vigorous sports activity and keeping your home free of clutter. Making an effort to slow down and becoming aware of your surroundings can also help.

With Aries' rulership of the head, there can be a tendency toward accidents to the head. By wearing a helmet when riding a bicycle or rollerblading, for example, you will cut down on the risk of a head injury if you fall. And it is just good common sense to wear a helmet when on a motorcycle or motor scooter.

Aries is a fire sign and, combined with the Sun, gives you good resistance to disease and a strong constitution. When illness occurs, it can be quick and severe but soon over. You tend toward inflammatory complaints and toward running a fever when ill, which is your body's way of burning off an infection. There can be an imbalance in your use of energy, and you need the attributes of your opposite sign, Libra, which include balance and moderation. You expect your energy to be unlimited and need to learn how to conserve it to avoid burnout. Eating peaches and pears helps balance the system. Your seemingly unlimited energy can benefit from a regular exercise regimen. This will keep your muscles toned and help you conserve energy. And as a fire sign, you are revitalized by pure sunlight.

With Aries' rulership of the brain combined with the vitality of the Sun, there can be mental exhaustion, which can be helped by herbs such as ginseng or valerian. The Sun in Aries makes the head area vulnerable, leading to such disorders as headaches, migraines, strokes, delirium, vertigo, high fever, eye problems, brain damage, concussions, and acne. Allowing yourself restful periods of relaxation can help prevent mental fatigue as well as headaches and migraines. Always have adequate light for reading and other close work to avoid eyestrain. Cutting down on sugary and fatty foods can help prevent acne. A healthy diet and a regular program of exercise are aids to good circulation and the prevention of strokes.

With the Sun in Aries, you are easily stimulated and can benefit from calming foods such as strawberries, mangos, and watermelon, proteins such as eggs, milk, and turkey, and chamomile tea. Overstimulating foods such as chocolate, colas, and coffee can have an adverse effect on health. Aries benefits from foods high in iron, such as apricots, raisins, black currants, beets, cherries, lentils, radishes, and spinach, and may have a stronger need for meat than other signs. Aries also benefits from dairy products, honey, nuts, sunflower seeds, sesame seeds, tomatoes, lemons, grapefruit, and celery.

Sun in Taurus

This is an earth sign, giving stamina, fortitude, and a strong body structure. You are finely attuned to the physical world and have a good sense of taste, touch, and smell. As an earth sign, you become rejuvenated when in contact with Mother Earth. Activities such as gardening or cooking with fresh herbs and vegetables bring you a sense of peace. You tend to be slow and deliberate in action to the point that you can become rigid and inflexible. Your body can become tense and subject to such disorders as constipation, rigid muscles, or arthritis. Increasing fiber in the diet can help prevent constipation. Avoiding refined foods and hydrogenated fats and increasing intake of fresh fruits and vegetables help prevent both constipation and arthritis. Eating cherries is also an aid to relief from arthritis.

You may clench your jaw when sleeping. You would benefit from stretching exercises or having massages. This will help your muscles and help give you a better night's sleep. Psychologically, you need to learn how to let go to keep from getting stuck in a rut.

Taurus is known to be a gourmand with a finely attuned palate. You may have a sweet tooth and tend to overindulge in rich or heavy foods. These food excesses can lead to anything from a stomach disorder to obesity, with the potential health risks caused by obesity. Obesity can create back problems, hypertension, heart disease, and diabetes. A reduction in rich foods and foods high in sugar and an increase in high-fiber and low-calorie vegetables can help you reduce weight. You might also try eating your largest meal early in the day, when you are able to burn more calories.

With the Sun in Taurus, you are vulnerable in the throat and neck area, the larynx, tonsils, adenoids, inner ears, gums, lower jaw, vocal cords, and thyroid. There can be throat inflammation. You may experience sore throats, tonsillitis, hoarseness, and dry coughs. There is the potential for goiter and glandular swellings. It is important to keep your neck covered during cold weather to avoid a chill, thus avoiding a potential throat disorder. Having a raw vegetable salad every day and massaging your gums can help prevent gum problems.

Herbs such as sage or fenugreek can be used for sore throats, and coltsfoot for hoarseness. Kelp is an aid to the thyroid, as are foods high in iodine, such as Swiss chard, watercress, broccoli, mushrooms, spinach, red cabbage, and potato skins. Spices such as parsley and oregano can help liven up the system, and root vegetables will help clean the digestive tract. Taurus has a love of routine and can get fixated on the same foods. You need roughage and variety in your diet.

Sun in Gemini

You are communicative, versatile, and mentally adept. You are easily bored, with a strong, inquisitive nature. Your need for constant mental stimulation can put a strain on the nervous system, causing you to be restless, nervous, and high-strung. You need periods of rest and relaxation and calming techniques such as meditation and yoga. Keeping your hands busy with such activities as knitting or sewing or even card playing can alleviate nervousness. Deep-breathing exercises and aerobic-type exercises can provide an outlet for your nervous energy. Dancing is also beneficial. It can be difficult for you to turn your mind off, and you should probably avoid mentally stimulating activities or foods high in caffeine at night. Any type of physical exercise that causes healthy fatigue helps your body and mind relax.

When ill, people with the Sun in Gemini tend toward nervous or respiratory disorders, allergies, and weak lungs. You are predisposed to diseases such as bronchitis, pneumonia, pleurisy, and asthma. Your breathing can be shallow and should be deepened to get proper oxygenation in the bloodstream. Drinking plenty of fluids and lowering your intake of dairy products can help ward off respiratory disorders. Vitamin B6, vitamin C, vitamin A, and zinc can also help prevent respiratory disorders. Keeping your home free of dust and avoiding the use of cleaning agents containing harsh chemicals can help prevent allergies. Ginseng powder added to herbal drinks can help ward off allergic attacks. Asthma sufferers may be allergic to milk, orange juice, fish, nuts, chocolate, butter, and peanut butter—substances to avoid if you are prone to asthma. Your lungs can benefit from garlic, flaxseed tea, wintergreen tea, and especially from vitamin E if you live in a smoggy area.

Carelessness can result in injuries to the arms and fingers, which need to be guarded, and you are also prone to disorders such as carpal tunnel syndrome, which can be alleviated by the use of acupressure and vitamin B6. You have a tendency to run on nervous energy and need to build up your muscles, which will help you gain strength and stamina. Gemini tends toward mental problems such as worry, anxiety, and hysteria and would benefit from positive thinking and calming herbs such as bergamot and skullcap. Gemini can benefit from vitamins A, B, C, and D to aid the lungs, flaxseed for coughs and bronchial complaints, and lemon balm for relaxation and sleep. A lavender pillow can aid sleep. Gemini responds positively to reflexology, massage, and aromatherapy, and chiropractic adjustment and osteopathy for shoulder pain. As an air sign, you can recharge yourself with fresh air, any kind of social involvement, and intellectual stimulation. You can be adversely affected by polluted air, and do well in the country or the mountains.

You need to eat a balanced diet with as many fruits and vegetables as possible, and you also benefit from eating nuts, green leafy vegetables, carrots, and cauliflower. Ginseng is an excellent body regulator. Dairy foods should be kept to a minimum, as they can be mucus-forming and can adversely affect your lungs.

Sun in Cancer

Cancer is a sign of nurturing and fluctuation. It is a water sign, which is considered the weakest of the four elements (fire, earth, air, water), as it is too easily receptive to outside stimuli. However, Cancer has great tenacity and has a strong hold on life. You have the ability to rebound from illness and usually become healthier as you get older. You are happiest when you are able to nurture and protect those you love and can easily become depressed if you do not feel you are giving or receiving enough love.

The Sun in Cancer has to come to terms with its strong emotional nature. Since the changeable and fast-moving Moon rules Cancer, you are subject to frequent mood swings and changing energy patterns. You have a tendency to worry, and, being a water sign, you can absorb negativity from those around you. It is necessary for you to psychically protect yourself from negative vibrations surrounding you, as you can easily absorb not only negativity but also toxins in the air. A healthy diet and positive emotional outlets are aids to good health. You can also mentally surround yourself with an invisible shield that deflects negative energy.

You need to learn how to discriminate between your feelings and the reality of a situation. Your overactive imagination causes you to perceive ailments that you do not have. Misuse of your emotions can lead to moodiness, irritability, and emotional upheaval and can drain your energy. Use your imagination in a positive way to see yourself as a vibrant, healthy individual.

You enjoy good food and large family gatherings at mealtime and tend to overeat. You are prone to weight problems, both from overeating and due to a tendency to retain water, which can be caused by a lack of potassium in the body or an imbalance of sodium. Excess fluid in the body can lead to swollen ankles. You could be helped by vitamin B6, alfalfa tablets, and the cell salt Natrum Muraticum. You would benefit from eating foods such as lima beans, endives, watercress, bananas, and avocados. Eating fish a few times a week is also beneficial. Lowering your intake of juicy fruits such as melons and increasing diuretic foods can help decrease water retention. Diuretic foods and herbs such as broom tea, celery, corn silk tea, grapes, juniper berries, raw onions, and parsley as well as weekly massages can help eliminate fluids in the body and break down fatty tissues.

The Sun in Cancer can indicate a weakness in the breast area, the rib cage, the stomach, and the entire alimentary canal. You tend toward digestive complaints, ailments such as arthritis and rheumatism, ulcers, and anemia. A combination of beet and carrot juice helps guard against anemia. You may experience stomach inflammation when upset, which can be helped by chamomile tea. The sign Cancer is associated with eating disorders that run the gamut from malnutrition to anorexia and bulimia. Having your Sun in Cancer does not mean you will get these eating disorders. Rather, the sign Cancer is part of an astrological signature for eating disorders.

Cancer's natural dislike of exercise can lead to flabbiness. There can be a weakness in the sinus cavities, gallbladder, chest cavity, and pleura of the lungs. You may also overindulge in dairy foods, which can lead to mucus formation in the body. Excess phlegm in the chest can lead to coughing. Thyme is a useful herb for eliminating phlegm and helping the lungs. Following good nutrition and adding two tablespoons a day of raw millet bran to juice or cereal help the gallbladder. Sage and slippery elm bark are aids to sinus disorders.

Women with the Sun in Cancer are prone to female problems such as bloating and swollen or tender breasts during the monthly cycle. These symptoms may be alleviated by cutting down on caffeine-rich foods, supplementing your diet with calcium and magnesium, and massaging with St. John's wort oil.

You are prone to stomach discomfort, which can be helped by papaya tablets, enzyme tablets, and lecithin. You should not eat when worried or anxious, as this can lead to digestive problems. Lettuce is a Cancer plant, which can soothe the stomach. You need to abide by a diet of natural foods and avoid overcooked foods that can ferment in the stomach and cause digestive problems. At each meal, you need to eat raw foods, which contain enzymes that aid your digestion.

As a water sign, you benefit from water therapies. Taking baths, going swimming or sailing, or relaxing by a body of water can recharge you.

Other useful remedies for the sign Cancer include the homeopathic remedy Nux Vom for stomach upsets and nervous indigestion, the herb arrowroot to calm the stomach, bilberry for water retention, cloves for stomach gas, and fenugreek tea to soothe an inflamed stomach.

Sun in Leo

The Sun has rulership over the sign Leo, strengthening its fiery nature and giving you vitality, endurance, and resistance to disease. You have the ability to bounce back quickly from illness. As a fire sign, you need to learn to pace yourself, as you tend to overexhaust your energy. Like your ruler, the Sun, which is at the center of our solar system, you also like to be the center of attention. You have much pride and can feel unwell when you do not feel you are getting enough notice or when you do not utilize your creative skills. You can find a healthy outlet in any activity that allows you to show off your creative abilities.

Leo is a fixed sign and does not take easily to change. A rigid attitude can affect the body in the form of stiff joints or muscles. When tense or depressed, you are prone to severe back pain. You should engage in activities such as yoga or stretching that encourage flexibility in the torso and back. It is important to learn proper ways of bending to avoid straining your back. Therapies such as the Alexander Technique can aid back and spinal problems. There can also be a rigid adherence to the same diet, which does not allow for a variety of foods containing sufficient vitamins and minerals.

Leo rules the muscular portion of the heart, giving you a warm heart and a generous nature. However, this is a sensitive part of the body, with a potential for cardiac troubles. Besides problems with the middle back, you are also susceptible to feverish conditions, heart palpitations, arrhythmia, chest pain, rheumatic fever, spinal problems, headaches, circulatory disorders, anemia, and hypertension. Cutting down on sugar and sodium and increasing the consumption of raw vegetables help prevent hypertension. A love of rich foods can increase cholesterol levels. Good nutrition is the first step in controlling heart disease and keeping the blood pure. Cutting down on sodium, red meats, and fatty foods, including soy products in your diet, eating plenty of legumes, and eating walnuts and seaweed products all help reduce the risk of heart disease. Obviously, not smoking and a sensible diet and exercise also aid in preventing heart disease. A combination of beet and carrot juice helps prevent anemia. Marigold tea is helpful for headaches.

Leo can be prone to sunstroke and high fevers or inflammatory disorders. Calendula cream, comfrey ointment,[1] apple cider vinegar, or witch hazel compresses help reduce inflammation in the body. Bee pollen and aloe vera are also helpful in preventing inflammation. You are also subject to eye inflammation. A good eyewash can be made by combining goldenseal tea with crushed fennel seed tea and boric acid and then straining the mixture.

Leo is associated with the vitality of the blood. Leo needs blood-strengthening foods such as red clover tea, borage tea, dandelion tea, wheatgrass, raw carrots and beets, black currants, raspberries, lemons, blackberries, blueberries, and watercress and must maintain purity of blood and see to proper elimination. You can also build up your blood with citrus fruits, raspberry leaf tea, and vitamins A, B, and C.

As a fire sign, you benefit from a moderate amount of sunshine every day. Leo can benefit from herbs such as angelica for heartburn, red clover as a tonic, motherwort as a heart tonic, and mustard to alleviate back pains. You should also avoid allowing too much heat to your back. Vitamin E and magnesium are also beneficial to Leo. Walnuts are a Leo food.

Sun in Virgo

Virgo is an earth sign with a practical bent and a strong interest in health but a tendency toward negative thinking and hypochondria. You can exhaust yourself by constant worrying or overworking, leading to nervous anxiety or intestinal disorders. Virgo loves to be of service to others and finds pleasure in a job well done. When unhappy, you become petty, overly critical, and anxious. You do not take well to criticism, can feel guilty for no reason, and can worry unnecessarily about your health, especially when given a health diagnosis. Since you are ruled by Mercury, the planet of the mind, you can alleviate anxiety by educating yourself on your health complaints and by practicing positive thinking.

You have good resistance to disease and the ability to assimilate and utilize food effectively. Your constitution is strengthened by keeping the bowels and nervous system in peak condition.

The sensitive parts of your body include the bowels, lungs, and nervous system. The intestines can be weak, leading to disorders and diseases such as duodenitis and peritonitis. Yogurt and buttermilk help fight disorders of the intestinal tract. Cabbage, cucumber, and grapefruit are good intestinal cleansers. Bee pollen is good for any inflammatory disorder of the intestines. As you are prone to bowel disorders, there can be problems with constipation, diarrhea, cramping, and gas, or more serious disorders such as colitis or irritable bowel syndrome. You have a strong need for fiber in your diet, such as that found in fresh fruits and vegetables and grains. Spinach is particularly helpful, as are alfalfa sprouts. Coriander tea can help dispel gas. With Virgo's rulership of the intestines, you are subject to forming polyps or having parasites. You may have food sensitivities, especially to gluten, and a tendency toward candida (fungus infection). A yeast-free, low-carbohydrate diet can help.

There can also be disorders of the liver and gallbladder, as well as respiratory and asthmatic complaints. Good nutrition is the key to preventing most liver and gallbladder disorders. Vitamin C, vitamin B6, vitamin A, and zinc help prevent respiratory disorders.

Virgo has rulership over the pancreas, and you are subject to disorders such as diabetes or hypoglycemia. You are more prone to diabetes if you are over forty, overweight, and have a family history of the disease. Gentle massage and exercise can help you. Good dietary habits and exercise help prevent hypoglycemia. Having breakfast every day and eating six small meals a day rather than three large meals will also help.

Your ruler, Mercury, also rules the nervous system. You have some tendency to be nervous and high-strung. Exercise can provide a healthy outlet for the nervous system. You tend to have strong dietary likes and dislikes. There may not be enough variety in your diet, which can lead to malnutrition. Artificial foods can be harmful to your system, and you do well on a diet of natural foods. Herbs beneficial to Virgo include balm and borage for nervous troubles, papaya leaf to stimulate the digestive tract, and skullcap to tone the nervous system.

Sun in Libra

This is the sign of balance and harmony, but your tendency toward indecisiveness and procrastination can lead to nervous exhaustion. You are healthy, with good resistance and recuperative abilities, as long as your body is kept in balance. This includes a life of moderation—a balanced diet and adequate rest and relaxation. You desire a peaceful environment and can easily become upset when placed in inharmonious surroundings. You will work hard to keep the peace. You function best in one-to-one relationships and can become physically ill when placed in a disharmonious relationship. This upsets your equilibrium, leading to lowered energy and emotional and physical problems.

Libra has rulership over the kidneys, which aid the balance of the body. The kidneys are responsible for the filtration and distribution of bodily fluids. The sign Libra is associated with body equilibrium. It is important that the sodium/potassium balance is kept in check. This balance can also become disturbed when you are upset or unhappy, leading to an acid/alkaline imbalance. Be careful of too many sweets and high-acid foods such as meat, soft drinks, and white pasta, as these can upset the balance in your body and lead to acidosis. Too much sugar and starch also increases acidity in the body. Keeping the system alkaline helps prevent gastrointestinal disorders and promotes good health. Lettuce, carrots, and celery help promote alkalinity. Keeping the body more alkaline also helps guard against infection.

People with the Sun in Libra have the potential for kidney disease, skin disease, headaches, and head and stomach disorders. There can be diseases caused by renal retention and the potential for skin irritation. Skin conditions can be helped by the mineral qualities of cucumber and the healing qualities of aloe vera. As you are prone to weakness in the kidney area, you benefit from drinking lots of water every day to keep the kidneys flushed. Herbs beneficial to Libra include cleavers and corn silk to promote kidney action, uva ursi for kidney weakness, feverfew to strengthen and cleanse the kidneys, and thyme for headaches. Kidney filtering is important, as it helps clear the blood of toxins. There can be lower back problems. The lumbar region is especially sensitive. Strengthening the abdominal muscles and lower back through exercises can help prevent lower back injury.

When nervous or unhappy, you are prone to skin eruptions, indigestion, and high blood pressure. You do not handle pressure well and are prone to adrenal exhaustion from stressful situations. Good nutrition and taking supplements such as magnesium and Siberian ginseng and herbs such as skullcap, vervain, and hops can help your body cope with stress. Physical exercise such as yoga, swimming, or walking can help alleviate headaches and tension.

Libra is ruled by Venus, a planet of relaxation and sociability. A day at a health spa or time spent in the company of congenial friends can recharge you. As an air sign, you are also recharged by fresh, circulating air and by plants that purify the air. Though you may crave foods high in sugar and starch, you need to eat plenty of foods containing sodium, potassium, magnesium, and iron.

Sun in Scorpio

This is a powerful sign that deals with the processes of elimination and procreation in the body. You have a strong constitution and the ability to resist and throw off disease. Scorpio is ruled by Pluto, the planet of transformation and regeneration. You are able to continually transform and regenerate your body by applying constructive health measures. You have a strong will and powerful emotions but a tendency toward extremes. This can be expressed as emotional highs and lows or a tendency toward drastic changes in your diet, leading to bodily imbalance. You are happiest when allowed to express your power potential and strong passion for life. When forced to submit to the will of another, you can easily become depressed, despondent, and resentful. A constant expression of negative emotions leads to mental and physical exhaustion. You need to learn detachment, or else you can develop psychosomatic illnesses.

People with the Sun in Scorpio are susceptible to diseases of the reproductive and eliminative organs. There is a sensitivity in the pelvic area and a potential weakness in the nose, throat, and tonsils. You are disposed to such disorders as nasal polyps or nasal catarrh, inguinal hernia, anal fistula, and hemorrhoids, and are prone to gastrourinary or bowel complaints. There can be inflammation and infection of the urinary bladder, as well as bowel disorders such as constipation or more serious disorders such as colitis or Crohn's disease. You need roughage in your diet on a daily basis. Fruits and vegetables and whole grains are a must. Herbs such as chicory and senna can be used as a laxative, witch hazel for hemorrhoids, and blessed thistle as a general tonic and to force out impurities in the body. Spinach juice and aloe vera are helpful to the colon. Parsley, watercress, celery, horseradish, asparagus, cucumber, potatoes, and watermelon help heal urinary tract infections.

Scorpio women are prone to uterine and ovary trouble and diseases such as cystitis and pelvic inflammatory disease. Bladder disorders can be helped by yarrow, witch hazel, juniper berries, goldenseal, and uva ursi teas. The ovaries can benefit from silicon and vitamin E. Men with the Sun in Scorpio can have a weakness in the prostate gland, resulting in an enlarged prostate or a difficulty in passing water. Zinc is essential for prostate health, and the consumption of pumpkin seeds is a good source. Tai chi and yoga breathing exercises are helpful for male reproductive health. Incontinence is a possibility for both sexes as you age. Cranberry juice taken in the mornings can help with incontinence. Bee pollen can be important in maintaining sexual health.

With Scorpio's association with the sexual organs, there is a need to guard against sexual excess to avoid sexually transmitted diseases such as gonorrhea or herpes. Needless to say, one should always practice safe sex. Scorpio is associated with the red blood corpuscles, which require iron. Foods high in iron include apples, beets, apricots, broccoli, blueberries, raisins, spinach, whole wheat, almonds, dates, and wheat germ. You need to keep your blood pure and can benefit from blood purifiers such as red clover tea and dandelion tea.

With the Sun in Scorpio, there is the possibility of a surgical operation at some time in your life. This could occur as the removal of your appendix.

A diet containing leeks, prunes, onions, beans, and barley will help energize you. You benefit from daily exercise such as walking, which will help prevent constipation and increase body flexibility.

Scorpio takes easily to drastic change, and when your health begins to decline, you are willing to make the changes necessary to improve health. You may benefit from acupuncture or acupressure and weekly massages

Sun in Sagittarius

This is a vital sign with much energy and resistance to disease but a tendency toward excess. You are optimistic and generous, which has a positive effect on your health. You are energetic and enthusiastic and need freedom to expand your horizons. When your activities are limited, you become unhappy and lose your sense of proportion, resulting in excessive eating and drinking. With your huge appetite, there is the potential for liver toxicity and increased uric acid in the body. There could be arthritic complaints in the hip joints and a tendency toward gout. A supervised juice fast helps clean out the liver. High-quality proteins, such as goat's milk, brewer's yeast, cottage cheese, and nut butters, aid liver function.

The sensitive areas of your body include the lungs, liver, hips, and thighs. You are prone to such disorders as sciatica, accidents around horses, locomotor diseases, and nervous ailments. Garlic and iodine are helpful against sciatica. The lungs are helped by flaxseed tea, comfrey,[2] wintergreen tea, and sufficient vitamin C. Thyme is also helpful for lung problems. Vitamin B is helpful for preventing nervous complaints, which can be exacerbated by alcohol. You enjoy sports, which are a good outlet for your fiery energy, but as a fire sign, you have a tendency to take risks, which can lead to accidents. You may also fail to recognize the limits of your body, leading to physical exhaustion. Exercises that strengthen the back help prevent sciatica.

There is a need to keep the blood pure, as there can be diseases caused by blood ailments. Your cholesterol levels can be high. Exercise and good nutrition can keep cholesterol in check. You may have poor lung capacity, which lowers your resistance to diseases such as pneumonia, bronchitis, and asthma. You need to avoid chills in cold weather and keep the chest warm. As a mutable sign, you are prone to mental and nervous strain. Older adults are prone to hip injuries and rheumatism and may need hip replacement surgery later in life. Rheumatism can be helped by cherries or cherry juice. You are prone to falls and should take proper precautions when walking on wet or icy sidewalks.

Your huge appetite can lead to obesity, and there is a need to moderate your food intake. You need to engage in physical activity, especially exercises that target the hips and thighs.

You benefit from an abundance of foods containing sodium, choline, iron, magnesium, and iodine. You should avoid foods that clog the liver, such as those that are high in fat or deep-fried. Herbs such as Oregon grape root can remove impurities from the liver. Dandelion is an aid to the liver and is a general tonic, and red clover is a good blood purifier. You can be helped by foods such as cucumbers to soothe the system, asparagus as a cleanser, and spices such as sage and cloves, which can be cleansing and stimulating.

Sun in Capricorn

You have a structurally sound constitution and much endurance. As an earth sign, you have a low vibration that improves with age. You are naturally disciplined, a follower of tradition, moderate, and prefer to live life at a slow pace. At times you can be demanding and inflexible, with a strong need to control your environment. You are happiest when in a position of authority, as when forced to bend to the will of others, you become overly rigid and obstinate. Loss of control also causes you to become depressed and anxious.

You have a tendency toward pessimism, which can lower your vitality. You can be stiff and uptight and need to learn to loosen up, as this rigidity and stiffness could lead to such ailments as rheumatism and arthritis. Engaging in activities such as swimming, stretching exercises, or deep-breathing exercises will help. Therapies such as reflexology and massage can be beneficial to prevent inhibition of movement and to help loosen up your stiff body.

You are susceptible to illnesses that begin with cold, which can lead to chills and aches and pains. Staying warm increases your resistance to illness. With Capricorn's association with the skin and bones, there can be inflammatory skin diseases and problems with the joints and bones. You are subject to dry skin and brittle nails, which can be caused by poor fat assimilation or a lack of animal fat. You benefit from an increase in healthy oils such as olive oil or canola oil. Massage has been found to be effective in dealing with musculoskeletal disorders. You should also be sure to stretch before and after vigorous exercise. You are prone to rashes and skin disorders such as warts and skin growths. A good nutritional program can guard against skin disorders. Apples and dark grape juice can help alleviate skin rashes. It may help to eliminate milk products, wheat products, coffee, and strong spices from your diet.

The knees are weak and should be guarded. You are subject to falls, bruising, digestive troubles involving the gallbladder, and lameness. Carrot, beet, and cucumber juice cleanse the gallbladder. You should have regular examinations by a dentist, as you are prone to dental problems. There can be thinning hair as you age and a tendency toward calcification or hardening of tissues. Yogurt and wheatgrass are helpful against calcification. Nettle and rosemary taken as a tea or used as a rinse can help thinning hair.

As an earth sign, you are regenerated when in touch with the earth and benefit from frequent nature trips such as a walk in a park or a trip to a national park. Herbs that are beneficial to Capricorn include bay oil for skin trouble, prickly ash for chills, chamomile and cloves for toothache, rose hips to retain flexibility of cartilage, and black willow for joint inflammation. Capricorn needs sufficient calcium to maintain bones and teeth. You should eat dairy foods such as yogurt or cheese for their calcium content. You also benefit from citrus fruits and nuts.

Sun in Aquarius

You have a strong constitution and the ability to resist disease. You are intellectually oriented and are constantly seeking the unusual. You are restless and utilize a lot of nervous energy. You are subject to nervous disorders and an uneven flow of energy in the body. You dislike conformity and are happiest when allowed to express your own individual nature. When forced to conform, you can become erratic and high-strung, with sudden mood swings, or you may experience a lack of coordination in the body. Aquarius rules the circulatory system, and you can be prone to such complaints as swollen ankles, high blood pressure, heartburn, leg cramps, blood poisoning, anemia, and heart palpitations. Circulatory complaints can range from varicose veins to phlebitis. Systems such as osteopathy are an aid to circulatory complaints. Onion and garlic are blood purifiers and aid circulation. Vitamin E and calcium are helpful for venous circulatory disorders. Circulatory disorders are worsened by smoking cigarettes.

You are prone to spasmodic troubles such as convulsions, fits, and epilepsy. Adequate intake of minerals, especially calcium and magnesium, is necessary. These also help calm the nerves. A lack of vitamin B6 and magnesium can contribute to spastic conditions, which are also helped by vitamin E. It is important to get regular eye checkups, as you are prone to eyestrain and other disorders of the eyes. There can be locomotor disorders such as a sprained or broken ankle. You are also subject to rare or unusual ailments.

You can be erratic in your eating habits, eating when the mood strikes or following fad diets that can cause a nutritional imbalance. You should try to avoid foods containing a lot of chemicals or heavily processed foods. Aquarius is involved in the oxygenation of the body, and as an air sign, you need to get plenty of fresh air to keep your body tuned. A trip to the mountains can be rejuvenating. Exercises such as walking, bicycling, yoga, and deep breathing are helpful. You also need a good night's sleep to recharge the nervous system.

Herbs such as passion flower can aid relaxation, prickly ash cleanses the bloodstream and is an aid in ankle sprains, rosemary used externally stimulates circulation, and valerian can quiet the nerves and be an aid for insomnia. Foods that have calming properties are recommended. These include strawberries, mangos, and watermelon, proteins such as eggs, milk, and turkey, and chamomile tea.

Sun in Pisces

You are highly sensitive and psychic, which can lead you to pick up negative vibrations around you and upset your emotional balance. You have strong creative urges and a desire to help others, and when these needs are denied, you become escapist and overly fanciful. You are prone to emotional disorders and physical illness of a nervous origin. Chamomile tea and valerian tea are aids against nervous attacks. Emotional disorders are sometimes linked to a deficiency of niacin. You are prone to environmental sensitivities and the negative effects of pollution. Vitamin E is an aid against a polluted environment. Overindulgence in food or drink can lead to water retention. You have a vivid imagination, which can lead to psychosomatic illnesses. There is a need to cultivate positive thinking. The lymphatic system is sensitive, and there can be a lowered immune response and swollen glands. With Pisces' rulership of the lymphatic system, you need to eat foods that build up the immune system and cut down on foods containing high amounts of white flour, white sugar, and too many refined products. Foods containing zinc and vitamins A, B, and C aid the immune system. Ample vitamin E, found in nuts, fresh wheat germ, cold-pressed oils, and stone-ground whole wheat products, aids the lymphatic system. You can build up resistance to disease with a healthy diet and the inclusion of herbs such as echinacea, thyme, rosemary, rose hips, and Siberian ginseng, as well as the natural healing agent propolis. Alcohol intake should be kept low.

You are susceptible to respiratory ailments, liver ailments, and blood disorders and can experience allergic reactions to common foods. Vitamin C, vitamin B6, vitamin A, and zinc help prevent respiratory disorders. Milk thistle is an aid to liver function. Common foods such as dairy products and wheat products can contribute to allergies. You are especially prone to allergies from seafood. You are highly sensitive to medicine, drugs, and alcohol, which can lead to allergic reactions. These allergic reactions can manifest as respiratory, skin, or stomach disorders. Vitamin C is an aid to preventing allergies. You can be negatively affected by stagnant air found inside office buildings. You are sensitive to atmospheric changes, which can have an adverse effect on your emotions. Illness can sometimes be due to a chemical imbalance in your body.

Your energy can vacillate, and you need foods rich in nutrients, as well as high-energy foods such as aged cheese, aged beef, carrot juice, strawberries, dates, cherries, prunes, liver, and spices such as ginger, cayenne, and garlic, to sustain you.

You are subject to sluggishness in the body and are prone to flabbiness and water retention. Your feet are especially sensitive, and there can be problems with the toes and heels and ailments such as corns and bunions. Foot pain can be helped by acupressure and massaging the soles of the feet. The feet benefit from reflexology. Tea tree oil and aloe vera gel can be used on corns and calluses. There can be intestinal disturbances and a tendency toward flatulence. Pantothenic acid helps with flatulence. The lungs can be weak, with a tendency toward mucus formation. Lemon juice helps prevent mucus formation, as does cutting down on dairy products.

With the Sun in Pisces, you are prone to diseases that are hard to diagnose or cure, as well as misdiagnosis. You need to get a second opinion on any health disorder. As a water sign, living near water, taking baths, or going swimming are aids to good health. Walking and meditation and quiet times of contemplation are especially beneficial.

You can benefit from ginseng as a tonic, chicory to eliminate mucus, and burdock root as a source of iron. Foods high in iron, such as liver, raisins, or dried apricots, are also beneficial to Pisces.

The Moon in the Signs

The Moon is the general ruler of the emotions, habits, family, and roots. In medical astrology it can describe your emotional responses, habit patterns that influence health, and functional disorders. Lunar disorders can involve fluids in the body as well as mucus and sweat. The Moon can describe your daily rhythms in relation to health and vitality. It rules change, and can make one more changeable and moody when in a water sign (Cancer, Scorpio, or Pisces) or in one of the mutable signs (Gemini, Sagittarius, Virgo, or Pisces). In women, it corresponds to the monthly cycle. The sign position of your Moon can indicate a sensitive part of the body and a proneness to illnesses related to that sign. Like the sign position of your Sun, the position of your Moon provides valuable information on potential vulnerabilities.

Moon in Aries

You are not one to dwell on your emotions, and are emotionally independent and impulsive, with a dislike of restriction. You can be high-strung, nervous, and edgy, especially when you feel your freedom of action is being curtailed. Good nutrition and magnesium supplements help you handle stress. You are subject to poor eyesight or eyestrain, disorders involving the head and face, and problems with the upper jaw and teeth. Your eyelids can become swollen. Any eye problems require a visit to the eye doctor. You can avoid eyestrain by using good lighting when reading and taking frequent breaks so as not to focus on one thing for long periods of time. Eyebright tea can be used as an eyewash or drunk as a tea to aid the eyes. Cucumber slices applied to closed eyes can also help with eyestrain.

There can be insomnia and headaches. Poor diet and allergies to foods such as red wine, papaya products, aged and sharp cheeses, and foods containing cheese can contribute to headaches. Supplements of vitamin B, calcium, and magnesium are helpful. A tendency toward sinusitis and catarrhal conditions of the ear and nose can be caused by a vitamin A deficiency. Sage and slippery elm bark, as well as citrus fruits, can help. You may also be subject to arthritic pains in your knees. Sea vegetables, cherries, cherry juice, watercress, wheatgrass, and garlic help prevent arthritis.

Women with this placement are subject to miscarriage during pregnancy. Pregnant women have increased nutritional needs and require higher amounts of protein, iron, and B vitamins. Needless to say, you should avoid alcohol during pregnancy and avoid excessive coffee consumption. Your doctor will advise you on salt intake, which has to be watched. You may benefit from supplements of vitamin B6 and magnesium.

Moon in Taurus

You desire comfort and security. Your emotions can be placid, and you are not easily riled. You have some tendency toward a rigid disposition and a dislike of change. This can make it difficult for you to rid yourself of bad habits that can adversely affect your health. You tend to get into ruts. You have a rich palate, with a tendency toward excess. The neck, ears, and throat are sensitive, and you can experience sore throats, nasal mucus, polyps in the throat region, problems with the Eustachian tubes, tonsillitis, and laryngitis. A healthy diet helps prevent ear disorders. A roasted onion applied hot to the ear can relieve ear pain. Sage tea is excellent for sore throats. There can be disorders involving the thyroid gland, and glandular swellings in the neck. Vitamin E and iodine as well as iodized salt aid the thyroid. The lower jaw and vocal cords are sensitive. The gums can be sensitive, with a tendency toward gum disease. Apples are excellent for stimulating the gums, and vitamin C is helpful in preventing periodontal disease. Applying goldenseal powder can help sore gums.

Moon in Gemini

Your Gemini Moon combines your intellect with your feelings, giving you a tendency to rationalize your emotions. You have a lot of nervous energy and enjoy being busy. You have a tendency to worry, leading to anxiety and nervousness. Soothing oils applied topically, such as lavender, geranium, and bergamot, can help calm frazzled nerves. Adequate intake of minerals, especially calcium and magnesium, also help calm the nerves. You are sensitive in the hands, arms, nervous system, and lungs. You are prone to asthma, lung catarrh, nervous disorders, and accidents involving the hands, arms, and shoulders. Herbs such as thyme and comfrey[3] are helpful to the lungs. Avoid spending too much time in damp or cold places, as this could increase susceptibility to lung disorders. Flaxseed tea can also be taken for lung troubles. There can be swellings in the tubes of the body. You have a tendency toward bronchial conditions and respiratory allergies, which can be helped by garlic, sunflower seeds, and fenugreek tea. You would benefit from deep breathing exercises and should avoid smoking. You need plenty of rest and sleep to recharge your nervous system and would also benefit from outdoor exercise such as long walks or hiking.

Moon in Cancer

You have a strong need for emotional security. You are sensitive and are prone to moodiness and emotional stress. Your health and vitality are dependent on your moods, and you can feel ill or overeat when emotionally distressed or depressed. Excessive food intake can also lead to obesity or gastric disorders. Eating more cultured foods such as sourdough bread, yogurt, and buttermilk can help digestive disorders. The breasts and womb are sensitive areas for women who may experience edema during the monthly cycle. Gynecological problems can be helped by red raspberry and herbs such as blessed thistle, uva ursi, and yarrow. Tincture of hawthorn, motherwort, or dandelion helps eliminate excess fluid in the body. The Moon in Cancer indicates a sensitivity in the chest area, upper lobes of the liver, diaphragm, and thoracic duct, and a potential water imbalance in the body. Eating high-quality proteins and foods such as goat's milk, raw and unsalted nuts and seeds, and nut butters aids liver function.

Moon in Leo

You have vitality, optimism, and a sense of pride. You are not one to dwell on your emotions, and rarely allow them to drag you down. You have a tendency to overestimate your abilities and can overstrain your body. The heart and back are sensitive areas, and when ill, you are prone to backaches, heartburn, fevers, inflammation, and high blood pressure. You can lower your chances for high blood pressure by avoiding caffeinated beverages and limiting your sodium intake. Cutting down on sugar and increasing calcium will also help. Apple cider vinegar compresses help relieve inflammation. Heartburn, which is caused by acid that escapes from your stomach into your throat, can be alleviated by techniques such as acupressure or drinking ginger tea. You may also be able to avoid heartburn by cutting down on proteins and consuming more carbohydrates at your evening meal. Leo is a fixed sign, and it can be difficult for you to break bad habits that can adversely affect your health. You desire rich foods, which can increase cholesterol levels in the body. To avoid backaches, you would benefit from exercises that involve bending and twisting to keep your spine supple.

Moon in Virgo

You have good recuperative powers and endurance but a tendency to obsess about trivialities. There can be an overconcern with health and a tendency to overmedicate yourself. Worry can be detrimental to your health, as you are prone to anxiety and nervousness. Some anxiety and nervousness can be caused by too much caffeine. Anxiety can be treated through therapy and behavior therapies such as biofeedback. There is a sensitivity in the intestinal area and a need to keep the bowels and digestive tract in good condition. There can be abdominal swellings and bowel disorders. Increasing fiber in your diet aids the bowels and digestive tract. A poor diet could cause blood sugar problems, leading to either diabetes or hypoglycemia. High-fiber foods also protect against diabetes. Eating six or more small meals a day and watching consumption of caffeine and sugar help prevent hypoglycemia. The liver is also a sensitive area. Apples and carrots as well as wheatgrass and aloe vera are helpful to the liver.

Moon in Libra

You have a good constitution, good vitality, and the ability to recuperate from disease. You work well in partnership with others and generally do not like confrontations, which can upset your emotional balance. There can be a weakness in the kidney function, which needs to be built up. There can be an inability to lose weight or edema in the hands and feet caused by weakened kidney action. Corn silk tea and pear juice are helpful to the kidneys. You may also experience lower back pain. Practicing good posture and getting sufficient exercise will help you avoid lower back problems. You are also subject to skin disorders involving swellings and abscesses. Some skin disorders could be caused by a malfunctioning kidney, which causes toxins to remain in the body. There is a need to keep your body in balance through regular exercise, good sleeping habits, and eating a balanced diet.

Moon in Scorpio

You have emotional intensity and a strong constitution but a tendency toward emotional extremes. This upsets the equilibrium of the body. You tend to overestimate yourself and, due to your compulsive nature, can get into ruts that are hard to climb out of. The Moon in Scorpio can indicate a weakness in the prostate in men and menstrual irregularities and a proneness to cystitis in women. Bladder disorders can be helped by yarrow, witch hazel, juniper berries, goldenseal, and uva ursi tea. Pumpkin seeds are a good source of zinc, which is essential for prostate health. The eliminative and reproductive areas are sensitive in both sexes, and there is danger of venereal infections in both sexes. You need to practice safe sex.

There can also be a sensitivity in the nasal cavity and diseases associated with the lower bowel and bladder. Adding barley to your diet improves both bowel and bladder functions. You are also subject to a hernia, which can be caused by a lack of tone in the body or a lack of magnesium. You need sufficient protein and vitamin C.

Moon in Sagittarius

You have vitality, good resistance to disease, and a positive outlook on life. You have a tendency toward exaggeration and overindulgence and a strong need for emotional freedom. You dislike restriction and are happiest when planning for the future. There is a sensitivity in the areas of the lungs, nervous system, and hips and thighs, and there can be diseases of the liver and blood and a tendency toward gout and sciatica. Garlic and iodine are helpful in preventing sciatica. Dandelion is cleansing to both the blood and the liver. There can be locomotor disorders, which limit your freedom of movement. The hips and thighs should be guarded during any sports activity and during the winter when walking on icy sidewalks. You tend toward shallow breathing and can benefit from diaphragmatic exercises, which aid the lungs.

Moon in Capricorn

You have endurance and a strong constitution but a tendency toward emotional repression and rigidity. You need to be in control, and dislike any authority but your own. A rigid disposition can lead to conditions such as arthritis and rheumatism, which can be helped by cherries or cherry juice. A Capricorn Moon indicates a sensitivity in the knees and a tendency toward skin eruptions, aching joints, dental problems, and stomach and digestive troubles. The gallbladder is particularly sensitive, so you should watch your fat intake. There can be bone ailments and swelling of knees. Physical exercise helps build up the bones. You can also benefit from dairy products such as yogurt, kefir, and buttermilk as well as foods high in minerals such as sea vegetables, whole grains, and cabbage. Regular visits to your dentist can help you avoid dental problems. You should also avoid foods high in sugar, which can cause skin eruptions. This combination of the Moon and Capricorn can cause a fluctuation in the water balance in your body. As you tend toward dryness, you need to drink sufficient water every day to maintain good health.

Moon in Aquarius

You have good recuperative powers and vitality. You have a strong sense of social responsibility and a need to feel unique. Your emotions are erratic, and you have frequent changes in mood. You can be nervous, easily excitable, and high-strung. There can be nervous troubles and hysteria. The herb rosemary helps alleviate and prevent hysterical outbursts and lifts your spirits. Herbs such as chamomile and passion flower have a calming effect on the nerves. The circulatory system is sensitive, and there is the potential for heart disease. You are prone to blood disorders such as anemia and blood poisoning. Red clover tea and parsley as well as the mineral magnesium are excellent blood purifiers. Vitamin C and carrot juice, or a combination of cucumber, spinach, and parsley juice, help build the blood and protect against anemia. Wheatgrass is also helpful. The eyes are sensitive, with the potential for eye problems such as cataracts and glaucoma. It is important to have yearly eye checkups. With the Moon ruling fluids and Aquarius ruling the ankles, you are prone to circulatory disorders, leading to swollen ankles and pain in the legs and a tendency toward varicose veins. Witch hazel, comfrey tea,[4] and lavender oil can be massaged on the ankles and legs. Cayenne pepper added to drinks during the day helps prevent varicose veins. You have some tendency toward psychosomatic illnesses, which can be helped by positive thinking.

Moon in Pisces

You tend to be emotionally sensitive and vulnerable. You have a strong need to dream and create and can have problems dealing with reality, which can lead to a dependence on alcohol or drugs. Your moods fluctuate, and there is a need for grounding. Heavy foods such as meat, potatoes, and root vegetables can help ground you. Your strong compassion and sensitivity to those in need make you an excellent worker in the healing fields. The immune system can be oversensitive, and there is a susceptibility to respiratory ailments. The lungs are weak, and there is the potential for diseases such as pneumonia or emphysema. You can build up your immune system with a healthy diet and the inclusion of herbs such as echinacea, thyme, rosemary, and rose hips. Thyme also aids the lungs, as do garlic and flaxseed tea. Your sensitive body makes you prone to allergies, especially from seafood. Vitamin C is an aid to preventing both allergies and respiratory disorders. Your highly developed imagination can lead to a tendency toward psychosomatic illnesses. You need to practice positive thinking.

Mercury in the Signs

Mercury is associated with the respiratory and nervous systems. It also affects speech, coordination, and mental afflictions. It can affect a sign in terms of a neurological disorder, mental disturbances, and/or the breathing process. Mercury's sign placement has an effect on one's thinking processes and agility. As Mercury is the body's messenger, its sign placement can affect hormonal activity in the body.

Mercury in Aries

You are an independent thinker, with much mental energy. Intensity in the thinking processes can lead to mental strain. It can be difficult for you to turn off your mind, leading to mental and nervous exhaustion and insomnia. You are prone to nervous headaches, vertigo, sleeplessness, and nerve disorders such as Bell's palsy. You benefit from calming foods such as celery, turkey, bananas, figs, chamomile tea, and valerian tea. The eyes can be weak, with a tendency toward astigmatism or dry eyes. Chamomile tea can also be used as a compress or eyewash for tired eyes.

Mercury in Taurus

You are serious and deliberate in speech and thought. You can be very stubborn and dislike taking advice, especially when it comes to your health. The neck and throat are sensitive areas. When stressed, you can experience hoarseness, dry cough, laryngitis, or a stiff neck. There can be a difficulty in swallowing. Sage tea is excellent for the throat. Coltsfoot tea as well as the use of honey can help with coughs. You need to chew your food properly to avoid choking on it.

Mercury in Gemini

You have a sound mind and are versatile and communicative but can be high-strung and have difficulty in turning off your mind at night. You need to practice relaxation techniques. You are good with your hands and can dispel a lot of nervous energy through crafts. You have a sensitive nervous system, are prone to respiratory disorders, and may experience allergies such as hay fever. You may be prone to asthma or pleurisy. Drinking plenty of fluids and lowering your intake of dairy products can help ward off respiratory disorders. Vitamin B6, vitamin C, vitamin A, and zinc can also help prevent respiratory disorders. Herbs such as coltsfoot tea, yellow dock, and ginseng can be effective against asthma. There can be nerve pains in the shoulders, arms, and hands. Rubbing fresh lemon on these areas can relieve nerve pain.

Mercury in Cancer

You are emotional in your thought and speech. You are attached to your ideas and become nervous and upset when challenged. You tend to worry unnecessarily. This can manifest as nervous indigestion, an acid stomach, or flatulence. You are prone to stomach cramps. You may need to avoid highly spiced foods and increase your intake of cultured foods, high-fiber foods, and salads. Peppermint tea can alleviate indigestion. You are susceptible to sinus problems. You think about food a great deal and look forward to each meal. You tend to overindulge in dairy products, which can cause phlegm in the system.

Mercury in Leo

You have much exuberance and can be dramatic and forceful in speech and writing. A tendency toward rigidity in thought can strain your body. You also have a tendency toward heart palpitations, fainting, backaches, nervous trembling, and mental fatigue.

Basil tea and carrot juice are excellent tonics for the body. It is important to take regular breaks from your work, such as walking or stretching, to avoid strain to the back.

Mercury in Virgo

You have a sharp, analytical mind but a tendency to worry too much, causing unnecessary anxiety. An overly nervous disposition can lead to bowel problems such as diarrhea or flatulence or more serious disorders such as colitis or diverticulitis. Making a tea of bruised anise or caraway seeds helps dispel flatulence. Treatment for diverticulitis includes avoiding seeds, fibers, and raw fruit until the condition improves. Peppermint tea helps with diarrhea, and aloe vera is helpful for colon disorders. There is a sensitivity in the intestinal region and a potential for blood sugar problems. You benefit from a diet high in fiber.

Mercury in Libra

You are bright and sociable but can be easily upset by inharmonious surroundings. You have difficulty making up your mind, which can lead to nervous anxiety. You are oversensitive to pain and may fear medical procedures. There can be nerve-related pain, vertigo, dizziness, and eye problems. Dizziness can be associated with anemia or high blood pressure, for which you need to see your doctor. It can be helped by silicon, a mineral that is found in foods such as greens, apples, cabbage, grapes, peas, peaches, strawberries, spinach, and walnuts. Catnip tea soothes the nerves and can provide relief from pain. There is the potential for urinary disorders, which can be helped by drinking cranberry juice, as well as skin complaints, which can sometimes be caused by coffee, cow's milk, strong spices, and refined sugar.

Mercury in Scorpio

You are sharp and critical, with a penetrating mind. A tendency toward compulsiveness and obstinacy can put a strain on your body. You can be an extremist in thinking, causing psychological disorders. Your neck may be subject to neuralgia, which may be caused by inadequate vitamin B1. You may experience disorders of the generative and eliminative organs. Women with this placement may experience a hormonal imbalance, leading to female disorders. Raspberry leaf tea is an excellent herb for women's disorders.

Mercury in Sagittarius

You are forthright in speech and consider yourself an expert on many subjects. You tend to ignore medical advice, as it is difficult for you to follow a prescribed routine. You are on the move a lot, enjoy sports, and can experience pain or injuries to the hips and thighs or conditions such as sciatica. Garlic and iodine are helpful against sciatica. Your lungs are sensitive, and you are prone to respiratory disorders such as asthma and bronchitis. Drinking plenty of fluids and lowering your intake of dairy products can help ward off respiratory disorders. Vitamin B6, vitamin C, vitamin A, and zinc can also help prevent respiratory disorders.

Mercury in Capricorn

You are a deliberate thinker, with the ability to structure your thoughts. Your tendency to be overly organized and strict can lead to stiffness in the body and ailments such as arthritis or joint pain. You are prone to knee disorders that involve pain, creakiness, or arthritis. There is also a proneness to rheumatism and gout. Cherries, fresh fruits and vegetable juices, parsley, alfalfa, and watercress are all helpful for these conditions. You may require dental work and need to do exercises to limber up your muscles. You may experience skin disorders such as psoriasis. It can be helpful to avoid yeast and wheat products and use goat's milk or soy milk instead of cow's milk to avoid skin disorders.

Mercury in Aquarius

You are unique and independent. You are progressive and willing to try unusual methods of healing. You can be erratic, nervous, and high-strung and subject to hysteria. You benefit from the use of calming herbs such as bergamot and skullcap. You may experience muscle cramping, pain in the calves or legs, fleeting pains throughout your body, and intestinal disorders. Rubbing on essence of cloves is helpful to relieve pain in the body. There can be circulatory disorders and nerve-related ailments. Systems such as osteopathy are an aid to circulatory complaints. Onions and garlic are blood purifiers and aid circulation. Calcium and magnesium are helpful in preventing nerve-related ailments. The combination of Mercury in Aquarius is also associated with speech defects, which can be helped by a speech therapist.

Mercury in Pisces

You are sensitive and intuitive and tend to learn by osmosis. You have a psychic sensitivity to your surroundings and can pick up negative vibrations around you. You tend to worry too much and dislike dealing with harsh reality. You can be vague, absent-minded, and prone to mental confusion. This can be helped by focusing the mind on one thing at a time and avoiding involvement in too many projects at once. Gotu kola and fo ti capsules (Chinese herbs) as well as ginseng and rosemary help the memory. There can be escapist tendencies such as watching too much television or using drugs or alcohol. Your feet are sensitive, especially to cold, and you may have corns, bunions, or flat feet. You are also prone to foot cramps. Foot pain can be helped by acupressure and massaging the soles of the feet. Tea tree oil and aloe vera gel can be used on corns and calluses. Nervous conditions can be caused by problems with sugar metabolism.

Venus in the Signs

Venus is associated with slackness and lack of tone. Its rulership of sugar and other sweets links it with disorders caused by excess. Its rulership of kidney action links it with kidney disorders and the resulting effects. Venus is also associated with the throat and thyroid gland. It has some tendency to relax and soften.

Venus in Aries

You may have a tendency toward skin eruptions on the face or more serious skin disorders such as eczema. Protein deficiency has been associated with eczema. Aloe vera gel and blackberry leaf tea can be used as topical applications to the skin. You are subject to eruptions of the scalp and a tendency toward dandruff. These can be helped by eliminating junk food and foods containing heavy plant oils such as palm and coconut from your diet. Eating nuts and seeds provides the body with oils that contribute to good health. Kidney dysfunction can lead to headaches, for which cold thyme tea is an aid. There can be gastric disturbances from consuming too many carbohydrates or rich foods.

Venus in Taurus

You are prone to disorders caused by excess. You have a sweet tooth, and overindulgence in sugary foods can play havoc with your blood sugar metabolism. You may be prone to rashes around your neck, swollen glands in the neck, infection in the mouth, and tonsillitis. A compress for swollen glands can be made with apple cider vinegar. The herb marshmallow will help against chest congestion and tonsillitis. Comfrey mouthwash, ointment, or tea bags[5] are helpful for conditions of the mouth. Physical and emotional stress can contribute to skin disorders or rashes. Good nutrition and the use of magnesium are preventive measures. The thyroid gland can malfunction. Kelp is an aid to the thyroid, as are foods high in iodine, such as Swiss chard, watercress, broccoli, mushrooms, spinach, red cabbage, and potato skins. Contracting mumps is also a possibility with Venus in Taurus.

Venus in Gemini

There can be weak pulmonary action and poor respiration. You are prone to asthma. There can be excess phlegm in the throat. Avoiding foods such as chocolate, milk, peanut butter, and nuts helps those prone to asthma or other respiratory conditions. Supplements of vitamin B6, vitamin C, and zinc are also helpful. Asthma responds well to acupuncture as well as fenugreek tea and aloe vera. Eating lentils is also helpful. Chest congestion and sore lungs are helped by applying eucalyptus oil to the chest area. Daily exercise on a stationary cycle can help increase respiratory capacity. Your sugar metabolism can be erratic, especially if you overindulge in sweets. You enjoy a variety of foods, which aids nutrition and balance in your body.

Venus in Cancer

You may experience stomach disorders from overeating. When upset, you are prone to nausea or vomiting. Drinking a combination of lemon juice and water each morning helps improve digestion. There can be a water imbalance in your body and disorders due to poor nutrition. Cutting down on salt and increasing the consumption of foods such as asparagus, corn, grapes, cucumber, and watermelon help release excess fluid in the body. You have a craving for sweets, which can upset your sugar metabolism. Females are subject to breast cysts and breast tenderness. Peach tea can be used to make a poultice to soothe the breasts. Steamed cabbage leaves can also be used as a compress for sore, tender breasts. Vitamin B complex, calcium, and magnesium along with the elimination of caffeine-rich foods can help reduce the occurrence of breast cysts.

Venus in Leo

You are subject to heart or circulatory disorders. The heart and circulation benefit from lemon juice. There is the potential for heart palpitations, spinal problems, backaches, and hardening of the arteries. A tea made from wild cherry bark or wild cherry syrup can help with nervous palpitations of the heart. Hawthorn is an excellent tonic for the heart. You have a tendency toward excessive consumption of rich and sugary foods, which can upset your sugar metabolism. Your fat intake should also be watched, especially the consumption of fried foods, to avoid hardening of the arteries. Garlic and onions help lower serum cholesterol. Acupressure and massage therapy are helpful in back and spinal problems. Yoga exercises can also strengthen the back.

Venus in Virgo

You are prone to intestinal disorders due to eating an improper diet or too much overcooked food. Bowel irregularities can be helped by consuming fresh fruits and vegetables and whole grains. A lack of variety in your diet and a craving for sweets can cause a nutritional imbalance. You may have a problem metabolizing sugar, so you should consume foods high in sugar in moderation.

Venus in Libra

You tend to overindulge in food and drink, leading to a nutritional imbalance. The kidneys are sensitive, and renal dysfunction can lead to skin disorders such as acne or eczema. Asparagus is excellent for stimulating the kidneys. Excessive sugar intake plays havoc with your sugar metabolism. It is important for you to eat a balanced diet and to live a rhythmic, balanced life. This can be achieved by establishing a regular schedule of eating and sleeping combined with physical exercise.

Venus in Scorpio

The eliminative and reproductive organs are vulnerable. There is danger of venereal diseases due to sexual excess. It is important for you to practice safe sex. Women with this placement may experience menstrual irregularities, and men can have a weakness in the prostate gland. Women benefit from consuming lemon juice, red raspberry tea, and lentils. Men should consume pumpkin seeds, sunflower seeds, and other foods high in zinc, which benefit the prostate. There can be throat problems and a potential for bladder disease. A weak bladder benefits from vitamins A and D, manganese, and potassium. Strawberry leaf and corn silk tea are also helpful. Onions and garlic help kill throat infections. Sage tea makes an excellent gargle.

Venus in Sagittarius

You have a rich palate, with a liking for fatty foods, which puts a strain on your liver and can also lead to skin ailments. You are prone to gout. Apples, carrots, and zucchini are helpful to the liver. There can be flabbiness due to lack of exercise. The hips and thighs are weak areas and would benefit from strengthening exercises. You are subject to increased mucus in the lungs. Fenugreek tea helps rid the body of mucus, as does lowering your intake of dairy products.

Venus in Capricorn

You have a tendency toward dry skin and hair, brittle nails, and skin irritation. The herb horsetail is an aid to healthy skin and nails, as is the mineral silicon. The herb nettles makes an excellent hair tonic. The knees are a vulnerable area and are subject to swelling. Marjoram, plantain, comfrey,[6] and apple cider vinegar can all be used in a compress for swollen knees. The kidney function can be weak, with the potential for kidney stones. Consuming cooked spinach can sometimes contribute to kidney stones. Cucumber, carrot, and beet juices help cleanse the kidneys. Magnesium helps prevent kidney stones. You have some tendency toward venous disorders such as varicose veins or phlebitis. Vitamin E and vitamin C are helpful in preventing phlebitis. You are also prone to bursitis in your knees. Calcium and phosphorus are helpful for bursitis, as is garlic.

Venus in Aquarius

You are prone to disorders of the blood due to poor blood circulation. This can lead to swollen ankles, cold extremities, or blood disorders such as anemia. Onions and garlic are blood purifiers and aid circulation. You are prone to disorders such as varicose veins. Vitamin C, vitamin E, and the B vitamins are important. There can be heart palpitations and an uneven kidney function. Herbs beneficial for the kidneys include corn silk and cleavers that promote kidney action, uva ursi for kidney weakness, and feverfew to strengthen and cleanse the kidneys. Wild cherry helps with nervous palpitations of the heart.

Venus in Pisces

Your feet are vulnerable and need to be kept warm. You are susceptible to corns and bunions, swollen feet, and lameness. Foot pain can be helped by acupressure and massaging the soles of the feet. Tea tree oil and aloe vera gel can be used on corns and calluses.

You have a tendency toward gout involving the feet as well as allergies due to environmental sensitivities. Carrots, celery, cucumbers, beet juice, and cherries are helpful for gout. Excessive alcohol intake puts a strain on your liver and should be used in moderation.

Mars in the Signs

The sign placement of Mars is considered to relate anatomically to a part of the body that is overworked or subject to infection, inflammation, irritation, or trauma. Its sign placement could indicate a part of the body that requires surgery or is subject to injury. Martian diseases usually involve fever, infection, and pain or are blood-related. They tend to be acute.

Mars in Aries

The head and brain are vulnerable areas. You are prone to mental strain, leading to headaches, pains in the head and eyes, and the potential for head injuries and cuts or blows to the head or face. Your head should be protected during sports activity to guard against injury. There can be skin disorders such as acne or ringworm, the potential for an aneurysm or stroke, itchy eyes, and possible eye infection or inflammation. Conjunctivitis is a possibility, especially if you wear contact lenses. Apis is a homeopathic remedy helpful for eyes that sting and burn. Placing cucumber slices over the eyelids helps with pink eye and eyestrain. Simple eye inflammation can be helped by eyebright tea bags used as a compress. Eyebright tea can be drunk as a tonic for the eyes. Any severe eye condition needs to be treated by a licensed eye doctor. Ringworm and other skin eruptions respond well to a wash of goldenseal tea. Eating garlic buds in a salad can help clear a headache.

You should always wear a hat when in direct sunlight, as you are susceptible to sunstroke and dehydration. With Libra being the polar opposite of Aries, there can be a tendency toward kidney irritation. You benefit from drinking lots of water every day to keep the kidneys flushed. Mars in Aries is a fighter, and this placement gives strength and endurance.

Mars in Taurus

The thyroid can be hyper, causing metabolic disorders. The throat area is vulnerable, resulting in potential difficulties such as polyps, adenoid ailments, laryngitis, boils on the neck, rheumatism in the neck muscles, and whiplash. Marshmallow root is an aid to the throat and tonsils and adenoid problems. Kelp is an aid to the thyroid, as are foods high in iodine, such as Swiss chard, watercress, broccoli, mushrooms, spinach, red cabbage, and potato skins. Lemon juice is beneficial for rheumatism. There can be bowel disturbances and, in men, an enlargement of the prostate gland. A diet high in fiber helps prevent bowel disturbances. Taking zinc and essential fatty acids such as flaxseed oil benefits the prostate. People with Mars in Taurus are also prone to contracting mumps and getting nosebleeds.

Mars in Gemini

This placement can indicate an overworked nervous system or nerve irritation, leading to disorders of the nervous system such as neuritis. You are prone to coughing, asthma, and rashes on the hands and arms. Valerian is a valuable nerve-easing plant. Vitamin B is important for nerve health. Celery is good for the nerves, and apples and carrots aid neuritis. The lungs are sensitive, and there is the potential for acute pneumonia, lung inflammation, or bronchial congestion. Smoking cigarettes is especially harmful, as you are prone to pulmonary emphysema. Garlic is helpful in lung disorders, as is wintergreen tea before retiring. Flaxseed tea, thyme, and comfrey[7] also aid the lungs. Women with this placement are subject to tubal pregnancy. The hands, arms, and shoulders are sensitive and subject to cuts, fractures, or wounds resulting from careless behavior.

Mars in Cancer

You have a sensitive stomach due to an overproduction of hydrochloric acid. Eating citrus fruit on an empty stomach or highly spiced foods can lead to stomach inflammation. You do not handle stress well, which can lead to nausea or vomiting. Emotional problems can lead to ulcers. Cinnamon oil, clove tea, fennel, and ginger are all helpful for stomach complaints. Licorice can inhibit gastric secretion and can help if you have a gastric ulcer. There can be rib cage abnormalities, and there is danger of injury to the ribs from an accident, so be sure to wear protective gear during sports activity. Your eyes are sensitive, and you are subject to swollen eyelids and conditions such as conjunctivitis. Cucumber slices placed over the eyelids help with pink eye and eyestrain. Simple eye inflammation can be alleviated by drinking eyebright tea. Women with this placement can experience miscarriage or abortion. Pregnant women need extra supplementation such as vitamin B6 and magnesium, octacosanol, vitamin C, and iron.

Mars in Leo

This placement can make the heart a sensitive organ. There is the potential for heart disease, heart palpitations, tachycardia, angina, pericarditis, endocarditis, and rheumatic fever. You need to consult a physician if you suspect you have a heart problem. However, there are tonic herbs for the heart such as hawthorn and rosemary, and consuming foods containing onions and garlic is also beneficial. With Leo's rulership of the back and spine, you are prone to back injury or backaches or muscular rheumatism of the back. The back benefits from good posture, vitamins D and E, and supplements that build up the bones such as magnesium, calcium, and manganese. Sunstroke is another possibility, so take proper precautions when in direct sunlight. Avoid too much heat to the back, as this can exacerbate a back condition. Mars in Leo gives energy and good recuperative ability.

Mars in Virgo

You have a tendency toward bowel inflammation, liver ailments, and a hyperfunctioning pancreas. Your overactive pancreas can lead to blood sugar problems. The liver and lungs are subject to infection. Dandelion root makes an excellent stimulant for the liver. Spinach and alfalfa sprouts aid the bowels. Flaxseed tea, thyme, and comfrey[8] aid the lungs. You are prone to disorders such as pancreatitis, gastroenteritis, peritonitis, and appendicitis. The ingestion of raw foods improves the action of the pancreas, helping prevent intestinal disorders and blood sugar problems. There can be flatulence in the abdomen due to poor digestion. Coriander tea is excellent for expelling gas. Dysentery can be a problem when traveling to exotic places, so you should avoid raw salads and peel the skin from fresh fruits before eating. You are prone to accidents in the workplace involving sharp tools, as well as sickness from overwork.

Mars in Libra

This placement tends toward kidney inflammation of a nephritic variety (pertaining to the kidneys), skin eruptions that are related to kidney dysfunction, and the potential for kidney infection. Itching and burning eyes as well as headaches may be associated with kidney dysfunction. Lemon juice is valuable for kidney and bladder infections. Asparagus helps stimulate kidney action. There can be bladder problems and a tendency toward lumbago (lower back pain) and shingles. Exercising regularly, taking vitamin C, and learning how to bend properly can help prevent lumbago. Pearl barley helps overcome urinary disorders. Adding cayenne pepper to the diet helps relieve the pain of shingles. Reducing stress through activities like yoga lowers the chances of contracting shingles. You are also prone to social diseases due to sexual excess, and need to practice safe sex.

Mars in Scorpio

This placement can indicate problems with the colon such as a spastic colon, an acid colon, hemorrhoids, and diseases such as pruritus (itching), colitis, and irritable bowel syndrome. Apples, figs, honey, licorice, and prunes all aid the colon. Bee pollen helps prevent hemorrhoids and pruritus. Urinary disorders are common with this placement. Men are prone to inflammation of the prostate, and women are subject to female disorders such as vaginitis, cystitis, and problems with menstrual flow. Raspberry leaf tea is an excellent women's herb. Zinc is essential for prostate health, and the consumption of pumpkin seeds is a good source. Both sexes are subject to diseases such as herpes or gonorrhea, which can be avoided by practicing safe sex. The throat is also a sensitive area, and there can be inflamed tonsils or larynx and throat problems. Herbs such as sage or fenugreek can be used for sore throats, and coltsfoot for hoarseness. You are subject to nosebleeds and should avoid blowing your nose too vigorously.

Mars in Sagittarius

You may be prone to injuries to the hips and thighs. There can be hip inflammation, sciatica, hip injury, or the need for hip-replacement surgery. You benefit from exercises that target the hips and thighs, which will strengthen those areas. Garlic and iodine are helpful against sciatica. Injuries to the hips and thighs can be prevented by wearing protective gear during sports activity and taking care when walking on wet or icy sidewalks. The lungs are sensitive, and there is the potential for pneumonia, bronchitis, and coughing spells. Vitamin B6, vitamin C, vitamin A, and zinc can help prevent respiratory disorders. Your nervous system is highly sensitive, creating a proneness to nerve-related diseases such as neuritis or neuralgia. Vitamin B is important for nerve health. Celery is good for the nerves, and apples and carrots aid neuritis. There is also the potential for injuries from horseback riding or being around horses. Mars in Sagittarius gives energy, endurance, and resistance to disease.

Mars in Capricorn

There is the potential for bruises in and around the knee joints, knee injuries, and inflammation of the knee joints. Marjoram, plantain, comfrey,[9] and apple cider vinegar can all be used in a compress for swollen knees and aching joints. You are subject to skin irritation, inflammatory and eruptive skin disorders such as psoriasis and eczema, and rashes. Good nutrition and possibly avoiding refined sugar, alcohol, coffee, strong spices, and cow's milk promote healthy skin and help prevent skin disorders. Drinking apple and dark grape juice helps alleviate skin rashes. The gallbladder is sensitive and there is the potential for gallbladder disease. You are prone to measles and mumps, rheumatic fever, broken bones, and gout in the knees. Drinking carrot juice before eating is good for the gallbladder. Carrot, beet, and cucumber juice cleanse the gallbladder and help prevent gout. Silicon is necessary for bone structure. Sage helps dissolve uric acid, which is a cause of gout.

Mars in Aquarius

This placement can indicate a potential for heart and circulatory disorders. There can be heart palpitations or valvular heart disease. A healthy diet and lifestyle changes such as more exercise, giving up cigarettes, losing weight, and controlling cholesterol levels can help prevent heart disease. Wild cherry tea helps nervous palpitations of the heart. You are prone to disorders of the veins such as varicose veins or phlebitis. Sufficient vitamin E is essential for healthy veins. The lower legs are sensitive and subject to rashes and breaks or sprains. Drinking apple and dark grape juice helps alleviate skin rashes. You are also subject to blood poisoning of the legs, ulcers on the legs, and back problems. Sufficient vitamin D and vitamin B6 can help prevent leg cramps and spasms. Onion and garlic are blood purifiers. The herb borage is a blood purifier.

Mars in Pisces

This placement can indicate a proneness to infections as well as weak vitality. You are subject to lymphatic conditions, sudden fevers, colds, flus, and respiratory disorders. There can be low blood calcium and blood disorders such as anemia. Supplements such as vitamins A, B, C, and E and magnesium and zinc help build up the immune system. Juices made from carrots, beets, lemons, oranges, green pepper, watercress, and parsley strengthen the immune system. The pancreas is sensitive, and you are subject to metabolic disorders involving sugar metabolism. Essential fatty acids are necessary for normal sugar metabolism. These include linoleic acid and vitamin E. A sensitive intestinal tract can lead to intestinal disorders or bowel inflammation. Chamomile tea, clove tea, and ginger tea all aid intestinal disorders. The feet are sensitive, with a tendency toward bunions, corns, or athlete's foot. Tea tree oil and aloe vera gel can be used externally for these ailments. There can be injury to the feet causing lameness as well as excessive perspiration or swelling of the feet. Sweat-inducing herbs include yarrow, chamomile, thyme, and hyssop. There can be adrenal insufficiency, especially when under stress. Good nutrition and the inclusion of magnesium help reduce stress. A drink made by juicing romaine lettuce with carrots stimulates the adrenals.

Jupiter in the Signs

Jupiter can be expansive, for better or worse. When stressed, it tends toward engorgement and a difficulty in fat assimilation. Jupiter generally has a protective nature but can indicate excess and immoderation. It is associated with liver dysfunction and blood diseases. The sign position of Jupiter can be associated anatomically with a larger-than-average part of the body.

Jupiter in Aries

You have excellent mental abilities and a good blood supply to the brain. There could be a tendency toward vertigo and headaches. Herbs such as peppermint, chamomile, ginger, and parsley help relieve headaches. Silicon is an aid to dizziness. The head can be larger than average. You may be prone to high blood pressure and in extreme cases stroke. Garlic has been helpful in treating high blood pressure. Cutting down on salt, sugar, and caffeinated beverages and increasing intake of raw vegetables help lower high blood pressure.

Jupiter in Taurus

You have a large appetite, which can lead to diseases caused by excess. There can be excess uric acid, leading to gout. Sage helps dissolve uric acid, which is a cause of gout. You are subject to enlarged adenoids or tonsils, dry coughing spells, sore throats, and an enlarged thyroid. There can be swelling in the neck. These disorders can be helped by apple cider vinegar, burdock, or fennel compresses to the throat, or by drinking sage tea. Ginseng helps as a glandular and body balancer.

Jupiter in Gemini

You have a tendency to be nervous and high-strung, with a sensitive nervous system. Yoga and stretching exercises can lower stress. Seawater baths and herbs such as chamomile and skullcap are beneficial. Your cholesterol levels should be watched, as there is the possibility of arterial disease. Supplements such as acidophilus, activated charcoal, and calcium can help lower cholesterol levels. The lungs are sensitive, with the potential for lung congestion, disorders such as bronchitis or pleurisy, or pneumonia. Thyme tea helps eliminate phlegm. You may also experience swelling in the hands and sciatica in the arms. Garlic and iodine are helpful in preventing sciatica.

Jupiter in Cancer

Your tendency to overeat can lead to weight gain. You are prone to gastric disorders, stomach upset, and flabby stomach muscles. You benefit from performing abdominal exercises to strengthen your stomach. You do better having small, frequent meals rather than three large meals a day. There can also be catarrhal conditions (mucus) and a tendency toward hiatus hernia. Fresh horseradish with lemon juice, fennel tea, or cayenne helps rid the body of mucus. A lack of tone in the body can contribute to hernia. The body needs sufficient protein, vitamin C, and magnesium to build up muscles and avoid rupture.

Jupiter in Leo

This combination can give a tendency toward blood disorders such as arteriosclerosis or circulatory problems leading to swollen ankles. A high fat intake could lead to heart disease. Garlic and onions aid heart action. Hawthorn berries make an excellent heart tonic. You may experience back pain. There can be high blood pressure and heart palpitations. Lemon juice and wild cherry bark extract are helpful for heart palpitations. Cutting down on salt, sugar, and caffeinated beverages and increasing intake of raw vegetables help lower high blood pressure.

Jupiter in Virgo

With this placement, the liver is vulnerable to problems such as enlargement, fatty degeneration, or cirrhosis. Alcohol intake should be kept to a minimum. Fat intake should be controlled to prevent excess cholesterol. Supplements such as whey, niacin, and vitamin A aid liver function. The bowels are sensitive, with a proneness to flatulence, diarrhea, or inflammation. Cinnamon and ginger are useful if you experience flatulence. Nutmeg and peppermint tea are useful in the case of diarrhea.

Jupiter in Libra

You may have a desire for foods high in sugar or fat, leading to problems in fat assimilation or glucose production. There can be weight gain and a tendency toward diabetes. Diabetes can be controlled by sensible eating. It is better to eat numerous small meals rather than three large ones a day, cut down on starchy foods, and increase essential fatty acids in your diet—sesame, sunflower, safflower, or flaxseed oil. There can be unsatisfactory adrenal and kidney activity. Blood impurities can lead to skin disease. A drink made by juicing romaine lettuce with carrots stimulates the adrenals. Red clover tea is a blood purifier. The kidneys are sensitive, and there can be cholesterol deposits in the kidney tubules or fever due to a disorder in the kidneys. Corn silk tea and pear juice promote kidney action.

Jupiter in Scorpio

You have good recuperative powers and resistance to infection. You are prone to diseases caused by excess, such as gout. Carrot, celery, cucumber, and beet juices are helpful against gout. There can be blood disorders such as blood poisoning and edema due to a water imbalance in the body. Tincture of hawthorn, motherwort, or dandelion helps eliminate excess fluid in the body. Comfrey is a blood cleanser and is also helpful against gout.[10] Men with this placement are prone to an enlarged prostate, and women are prone to inflammation of the womb. Homeopathic remedies such as belladonna and cantharis will help this female disorder. Pumpkin seeds and supplementation with zinc and magnesium are helpful to the prostate.

Jupiter in Sagittarius

This combination is associated with pains or swelling in the hips or thighs and a tendency toward diseases such as gout, rheumatism, sciatica, and high blood pressure. Garlic and iodine are helpful against sciatica. Lavender lotion or castor oil packs aid pain and swelling. Cranberry juice is an aid against gout and rheumatism. Cutting down on salt, sugar, and caffeinated beverages and increasing intake of raw vegetables help lower high blood pressure. There can be problems in fat assimilation, which put a strain on the liver. Dandelion is an excellent cleansing tonic for the liver. There can be ulcers on the hips and thighs. This placement indicates that excess weight can fall on your hips or thighs, so you benefit from exercises that tone these areas.

Jupiter in Capricorn

You are sensitive around the knees, which are subject to swelling or inflammation. Apple cider vinegar compresses help relieve swelling and inflammation. There is the potential for liver or gallbladder disorders. Cholesterol levels can be higher than normal. Cutting down on whole milk products can reduce cholesterol levels and improve gallbladder action. Taking two tablespoons daily of either raw miller's bran or oat bran improves gallbladder action. Good nutrition and including foods such as raw nuts and seeds aid the liver. You are prone to digestive ailments due to overeating. There can be skin diseases such as eczema or psoriasis. Cutting down on rich and oily foods helps prevent skin disorders and improves digestion.

Jupiter in Aquarius

You are prone to circulatory disorders that can lead to swollen ankles or more serious ailments such as varicose veins. Manganese helps protect blood vessels. The blood is aided by carrot juice. Blood poisoning is a potential, as is a spasm condition in the legs. Diluted lemonade with no sugar is a good blood purifier. Adequate intake of minerals, especially calcium and magnesium, is necessary to prevent spasms. There can be heart palpitations and high blood pressure. Garlic is helpful for high blood pressure. Rosemary is a quieting tonic for the heart. Red clover tea is helpful for heart palpitations. The back is sensitive and subject to swelling. Adequate calcium in the diet is necessary to prevent back problems.

Jupiter in Pisces

You have a sensitive immune system and are prone to colds and infections. Grapefruit is excellent for fighting colds. Garlic can help. You have a tendency toward swollen feet or lameness, which can benefit from foot massage. There may be disorders with the sugar metabolism in your body and a proneness to diabetes or hypoglycemia. Vitamin C, vitamin E, chromium, and niacin can help control diabetes. Hypoglycemia can be prevented by eating breakfast regularly, controlling sodium and sugar intake, and consuming more vegetables and beans. You are prone to edema and allergies to gases or fumes. Corn silk tea is an effective diuretic.

Saturn in the Signs

The sign placement of Saturn in your chart can indicate a weak organ or weak area of the body. This area of the body may not get a good blood supply and therefore needs to be built up or nourished. Since the signs work in polarity with each other, you may sometimes find that the sign opposite the sign of your Saturn is also a weak point in the body. The signs and their opposites are as follows:

Aries is opposite Libra.

Taurus is opposite Scorpio.

Gemini is opposite Sagittarius.

Cancer is opposite Capricorn.

Leo is opposite Aquarius.

Virgo is opposite Pisces.

Suggestions on how to build up and nourish these weak parts of the body will be given here and in appendix A. When you are ill, you may find that the sign occupied by Saturn or the opposite sign is where disease manifests. Therefore, you should also read the information on the sign opposite your natal Saturn.

Saturn in Aries

There is a weakness in the head area, which includes the hair, eyes, teeth, and face. Women may experience thinning hair and men may experience baldness as they age. Sage tea can help stimulate hair growth. Silicea, a homeopathic remedy, and foods containing silicon are helpful for persons with Saturn in Aries for most of the potential problems and weaknesses. Silicon is found in asparagus, alfalfa, all greens, oats, peas, rye bread, shredded wheat, strawberries, spinach, walnuts, and whole wheat. The herb horsetail is helpful for the hair and nails. The teeth are sensitive; there can be dental problems. There could be tartar or build-up of plaque, requiring regular visits to the dentist for cleaning. You are also prone to tooth decay and frequent cavities, which can be exacerbated by foods high in sugar. With Saturn's association with the bones, there is also the potential for periodontal problems such as bone loss or large pockets in the gums. Aries rules the upper jaw, which is another potential area of weakness. Vitamin D is necessary for bone formation.

Other disorders with Saturn in Aries include hearing problems such as mucus build-up in the ears, resulting in earaches and deafness. Hearing problems benefit from more vitamin C. Hops is good for earaches. Saturn in Aries can also indicate weakened adrenal gland function, which can result in a proneness to infection or poor resistance to disease. Vitamin C and parsley will help the adrenals. With Aries opposite the Libra-ruled kidneys, there can be weakened kidney function, which could manifest as headaches or skin irritation. Corn silk tea and pear juice promote kidney action. The eyes can be weak with Saturn in Aries, leading to nearsightedness, astigmatism, or cataracts. You need regular eye exams, as there is the potential for glaucoma. The eyes can be helped by vitamin B-complex, fennel, and a juice made up of carrots, parsley, and celery. You may also experience mental fatigue or listlessness because of a lack of blood supply to the brain. Lying on a slant board can stimulate the head area. You are prone to skin irritation, which could be caused by an allergic reaction to a face cream or cosmetic.

Saturn in Taurus

There can be a weakness in the neck and throat. At some point, the tonsils may atrophy and have to be removed. You may experience a dry cough, frequent sore throats, or more serious disorders such as whooping cough. You may find that you become hoarse or lose your voice when you become ill. There is a tendency toward phlegm in the throat, with the potential for polyps in the throat. Sage is good for the throat and for head congestion. Onions and garlic are good for a throat infection. Tonsils benefit from gargling with a chlorophyll liquid concentrate. There is the danger of choking on food while eating, so you should be sure to chew your food thoroughly before swallowing.

Taurus is involved with endurance and support in the body. Therefore, the gums, which are ruled by Taurus, can be weak with Saturn in Taurus. There can be bleeding gums, a tendency toward pyorrhea, or periodontal problems. You may need root canal work at some point in your life. Vitamins B and C are important for the gums. Raw cabbage and carrot juice cleanse the gums. With Taurus opposite Scorpio, which rules the colon, there is a tendency for bowel disorders such as constipation or diarrhea. Adding more fiber to the diet can help. Prunes, figs, and raw spinach salad can also help. The thyroid is ruled by Taurus, so this Saturn placement can contribute to a hypofunctioning thyroid or weakened thyroid function. Kelp is an aid to the thyroid, as are foods high in iodine, such as Swiss chard, watercress, broccoli, mushrooms, spinach, red cabbage, and potato skins. You are also prone to whiplash and neckache. You benefit from exercises that add flexibility to the neck muscles.

Saturn in Gemini

This placement can indicate poor oxygen capacity in the lungs or lung ailments caused by smoking, such as emphysema. Stopping smoking or doing deep-breathing exercises will improve lung capacity. Saturn in Gemini is prone to respiratory disorders such as bronchitis or lung congestion, and more serious disorders such as asthma, pneumonia, or tuberculosis. Garlic is helpful in lung disorders, as is wintergreen tea before retiring. Flaxseed tea, thyme, and comfrey[11] also nourish the lungs. Being in a damp atmosphere can contribute to respiratory disorders.

With the Gemini rulership of the arms and shoulders, there is a tendency toward rheumatism or arthritis of the arms, hands, or shoulders. You are also subject to blocked tubes in the body, fractures, and diseases that affect the arms and shoulders. Stiff joints can be bathed in sage tea. Grapefruit, apples, and carrots are aids for arthritic complaints. Magnesium keeps joints flexible. There is also the potential for fractures of the wrist, a dislocated shoulder, and disorders caused by repetitive motion, such as carpal tunnel syndrome. These can be helped by the use of acupressure and vitamin B6. Poor oxygenation can lead to a susceptibility to heavy metal poisoning from a polluted atmosphere, weak respiratory function, or pleurisy. Vitamin B6, vitamin C, vitamin A, and zinc can help prevent respiratory disorders. Food sources of oxygen include apples, cane sugar, grapes, green onions, limes, lemons, melons, and tomatoes. If you live in a highly polluted area, you could benefit from increased vitamin C, vitamin E, and vitamin D. Your nervous system is sensitive, and there can be nervous trembling from a lack of calcium and manganese.

Saturn in Cancer

This placement can indicate low hydrochloric acid levels in the stomach, causing poor digestive processes and gastric complaints. This combination is sometimes indicative of a lack of appetite and poor nutrition. Saturn in Cancer is part of a signature for anorexia and bulimia. With this placement, vitamins and minerals may not be absorbed adequately in the body. You should avoid drinking citrus juice on an empty stomach, as this can irritate your stomach. Raw dandelion is good for a hyperactive stomach. Catnip tea helps reduce stomach acid. Marjoram and chamomile are good for indigestion. Anemia can be brought on because the intrinsic factor (an enzyme produced in the stomach) is hyperfunctioning. You benefit from eating foods high in vitamin B12, such as beef, liver, eggs, milk, and cheese. Foods high in iron, such as apples, beets, apricots, broccoli, blueberries, raisins, spinach, whole wheat, almonds, dates, and wheat germ, are beneficial.

With Saturn in Cancer, there is a need to build up your digestive functions. There are different measures you can take to stimulate your stomach. Grapefruit juice acts as a stimulus, but it should not be taken on an empty stomach. Drinking cold water before a meal is also a stimulus to the stomach. If you do not have an excess of fire in your chart, you would benefit from increasing your intake of spicy food to help stimulate your stomach. This includes foods containing spices such as ginger or curry. Refrain from eating late at night, as your stomach doesn't have time to empty properly, causing you to wake up feeling bloated and tired.

Women with this placement are prone to breast cysts or fibroid tumors. Kelp can help the breasts. Women may benefit from taking the herb vitex, also called chasteberry. In both sexes, the ribs are a sensitive area and should be protected in sports activity. There can also be a tendency toward arthritis, stiff knee joints, gallstones, or sinusitis. Taking two tablespoons daily of either raw miller's bran or oat bran improves gallbladder action. Cherries, fresh fruit and vegetable juices, parsley, alfalfa, and watercress are all helpful for arthritic complaints and joint pain.

Saturn in Leo

This placement indicates a weakness in the heart and back. There can be weak muscular action of the heart, resulting in a lazy heart or weakened heart action. People with Saturn in Leo do better when involved in physical activity, and should avoid being too sedentary. There is a potential for hardening of the arteries, and cholesterol levels should be checked. Supplements such as acidophilus, activated charcoal, and calcium can help lower cholesterol levels. With the Leo polarity to Aquarius, there is the potential for circulatory disorders or constriction of arteries or veins leading to the heart. Manganese helps protect blood vessels. There can be swollen ankles from valvular heart trouble. Witch hazel, comfrey tea,[12] and lavender oil can be massaged on the ankles. Leo also rules the middle back and spine, so you may have backaches when under stress or be prone to spinal problems such as arthritis of the spine or back injuries. You would benefit from exercises that involve bending and twisting to keep your spine supple. You should also learn proper ways of bending.

Saturn in Virgo

This placement can result in intestinal blockage or constriction of the intestines. There can be bowel disorders and poor peristaltic motion, leading to either diarrhea or constipation or bowel to disorders such as colitis or irritable bowel syndrome. Herbs that are helpful include raspberry leaves, peppermint tea, licorice, aloe vera, and psyllium seed husks. You may have problems metabolizing sugar and carbohydrates due to a lack of enzyme production. Virgo rules the pancreas, and with Saturn in Virgo there can be problems with glucose production leading to disorders such as hypoglycemia or diabetes. Vitamin C, vitamin E, chromium, and niacin can help control diabetes. Hypoglycemia can be prevented by having breakfast regularly, controlling sodium and sugar intake, and eating more vegetables and beans. There is the potential for poor enzyme action within the liver. You need some build-up of the enzyme formation, which is best found in raw foods, especially raw pineapple and papaya. The intestines can also be stimulated by exercising, adding more roughage to your diet, including yogurt and buttermilk in your diet, and lowering intake of vinegar. Avoid consuming too much white sugar. Saturn in Virgo does not digest sugar or carbohydrates well.

Saturn in Libra

This placement indicates a potential weakness in the kidneys. There can be weak or sluggish kidney function or hypofunctioning kidneys, thickening of the tubule walls of the kidneys, and poor filtering conditions to remove urea from the blood. Saturn in Libra can indicate the suppression or scarcity of urine. This placement can also contribute to arthritic nodules or rheumatism. There can be back pressure from obstructed kidneys and the potential for kidney stones. These problems can be helped by lowering your intake of high-fat foods, milk, and milk products and increasing your intake of high-fiber foods. Magnesium helps prevent kidney stones. Eye problems or skin eruptions may be related to kidney dysfunction. Distilled water can be used as a diuretic to flush out the kidneys. You are also prone to pains in the knees and have a tendency toward gout. Marjoram, plantain, comfrey,[13] and apple cider vinegar can all be used in a compress for swollen or painful knees. Cranberry juice and cherries help alleviate the symptoms of gout. Adrenal function can be suppressed. The adrenals benefit from pantothenic acid.

Saturn in Scorpio

This placement indicates potential weaknesses in the eliminative and reproductive organs. There can be colon stasis, stones in the bladder, retention of urine, bladder problems, sluggish peristalsis, and a tendency toward hemorrhoids or constipation. You can benefit from figs, prunes, licorice, raw spinach salad, strawberries, and apples for eliminative disorders. Pearl barley helps overcome urinary disorders. In males, there can be weakened prostate function, an enlarged prostate, or low sperm count. In females, there can be weakness in the female organs. Pumpkin seeds and supplementation with zinc and magnesium are helpful to the prostate. Bee pollen is also helpful for prostate health. Raspberry leaf tea is a tonic for women. With reflex action to Taurus, the sign opposite Scorpio, you may also find that the throat region is vulnerable, resulting in throat problems, phlegm, hoarseness, and poor thyroid defense. Kelp is an aid to the thyroid, as are foods high in iodine, such as Swiss chard, watercress, broccoli, mushrooms, spinach, red cabbage, and potato skins. Herbs such as sage or fenugreek can be used for sore throats, and coltsfoot for hoarseness.

Saturn in Sagittarius

This placement indicates a potential weakness in the hip and thigh region. There can be chronic sciatica problems, hip-joint disease, and the need for a hip replacement. Garlic and iodine are helpful against sciatica. You may be prone to locomotor disorders. Saturn in Sagittarius indicates poor lung capacity, leading to such conditions as bronchitis, and weakness in the diaphragm, causing problems with inhalation. The exhalation of breath can be shallow, which can be helped by deep-breathing exercises. Vitamin A and vitamin E are needed for healthy breathing. Wild cherry and coltsfoot help against bronchitis. Lung conditions can be exacerbated by smoking or dampness. Clove oil makes a good expectorant for lung disorders. You may have a tendency toward high protein or alcohol intake, leading to conditions such as gout. You are also vulnerable to tuberculosis and accidents to the hips and thighs. You need to wear protective gear when involved in any vigorous activity to avoid injuries to the hips and thighs. The nervous system is also sensitive, and you are prone to nervous disorders. Chamomile tea and clove tea help quiet the nerves.

Saturn in Capricorn

This placement can indicate a sluggish gallbladder and the potential for gallstones. A hyperfunctioning gallbladder can lead to inadequate bowel function and the release of too little bile from the gallbladder, resulting in bowel toxicity and digestive problems. Carrot, beet, and cucumber juice cleanse the gallbladder. Dandelion is a good remedy for gallstones. The digestion can also be weak due to an obstruction in the flow of gastric juices and a lack of hydrochloric acid in the stomach. The knees are a weak area and can become stiff or arthritic. You may be prone to rheumatism and stiffness in the body and have problems with the skin and bones. There can be dry skin or more serious skin diseases such as psoriasis or eczema. There can also be arteriosclerosis due to excess cholesterol. Supplements such as acidophilus, activated charcoal, and calcium can help lower cholesterol levels. Foods high in pectin help reduce blood cholesterol levels. These include fresh fruits, especially raw apples. Cherries and cherry juice help alleviate arthritic symptoms. Silicon is an aid for the skin and bones.

Saturn in Aquarius

This placement can indicate poor circulation, with a tendency toward cold extremities. Rosemary is an aid to sluggish circulation. There is poor oxidation, causing a lack of oxygen in the blood, and the potential for carbon dioxide retention. This can lead to iron deficiency. Food sources of oxygen include apples, cane sugar, grapes, green onions, limes, lemons, melons, and tomatoes. Iron is found in foods such as beet greens, molasses, nuts, carrots, cabbage, and raisins. You are susceptible to carbon monoxide poisoning and should have a device for detecting carbon monoxide in your home. You may also experience muscle cramping in the lower legs, a sprained ankle or weak ankles, or a weakness in the lower legs. Arnica ointment is excellent for muscle cramps or spasms, as is eucalyptus oil or a compress of apple cider vinegar. Spinal problems are a possibility with Saturn in Aquarius. A healthy spine needs calcium, magnesium, silicon, and vitamin B12. You need to practice good posture and do exercises that strengthen the back. There can also be eye problems, as there can be a poor blood supply to the retina and the potential for cataracts. Borage tea helps strengthen the eyes. The combination of Saturn in Aquarius shows up in cases of clubfoot and spinal curvature. Arteriosclerosis is also a possibility, as Aquarius is opposite Leo, making the heart and circulation weak areas. Calcium strengthens the arteries. Carrots, garlic, and pineapple juice aid the arteries. Chlorophyll liquid is a treatment for arteriosclerosis. Pectin is also an aid.

Saturn in Pisces

There can be a deficiency in the immune system caused by a low white blood cell count. You may have vitality problems or get frequent colds. Grapefruit is excellent for fighting colds. Juices containing carrots, garlic, black currants, oranges, beets, green peppers, or watercress help build the immune system. Pisces rules the feet, so this placement can indicate fallen arches, deformed feet, a tendency toward cold feet, or injury to the feet. There can also be arthritis or gout in the feet. It is important for you to keep your feet warm, as this will help to prevent colds. There is the potential for bunions and corns. Acupressure can help foot pain. Massaging the soles also helps the feet. Tea tree oil and aloe vera gel soothe the feet. With reflex action to the opposite sign of Virgo, there can be a weak pancreas and sugar problems. Essential fatty acids are necessary for normal sugar metabolism. These include linoleic acid and vitamin E. The liver is sensitive, and there can be sluggish action and poor filtering by the liver. Good nutrition and including foods such as raw nuts and seeds in the diet aid the liver. Worry is common with Saturn in Pisces, and cultivating a more positive attitude aids the immune system.

The Outer Planets

The planets Uranus, Neptune, and Pluto are called the outer planets, or the modern planets, as they were not discovered until the invention of the telescope. They move much more slowly than the other planets and can be referred to as generational planets, as they can describe the social changes of an entire generation. They work in tandem with the other planets and provide useful information in terms of health. Like the other planets, their effects can be for better or worse depending on how they are configured in the chart. The sign tenancy of each of the outer planets should not be judged alone. They work in combination with the rest of the birth chart to repeat or emphasize a particular theme. For example, if the birth chart shows a propensity toward headaches, having Uranus in Aries would be one more confirmation of this. But to read Uranus in Aries, or any of the sign placements of the outer planets, as an indication of a particular health problem would be erroneous, as the sign placements of the outer planets affect generations more than individuals.

Uranus in the Signs

The effect of Uranus is to describe a part of the body that can be subject to sudden disorders, spasm, surgery, incoordination, ruptures, or cramps.

Uranus in Aries

This placement can indicate spasmodic kidney action. Corn silk tea and pear juice promote kidney action. There can be spasm conditions in the face and disorders such as Bell's palsy as well as fluctuation problems in vision. A lack of vitamin E, magnesium, and vitamin B6 can lead to spastic conditions. You may also experience spasmodic headaches and eyestrain. There can be shooting pains in the head, sudden headaches, pain in the eyes, or a spastic condition of the blood vessels of the eye. Borage tea strengthens the eyes, and cucumber slices or a compress of chamomile tea soothe the eyes and relieve eyestrain. A fennel tea wash also helps the eyes. Peppermint, rosemary, and sage teas help alleviate headaches.

Uranus in Taurus

This placement can indicate a spastic condition in the thyroid gland, causing it to go from hyper to hypo functioning. A tendency toward nervousness could be caused by a malfunctioning thyroid gland. Kelp is an aid to the thyroid, as are foods high in iodine, such as Swiss chard, watercress, broccoli, mushrooms, spinach, red cabbage, and potato skins. There can be sudden attacks of laryngitis and the potential to choke or gag on food. A combination of lemon juice, honey, and a pinch of cayenne pepper will help with laryngitis. You are susceptible to loud noises, which can cause you severe discomfort. Mullein oil makes an excellent earache oil. You are also susceptible to a spastic colon. During any flare-up, you need to eat easy-to-digest foods such as rice, sweet potatoes, steamed vegetables, and bananas.

Uranus in Gemini

There can be a potential for cramps and spasms in the hands, arms, or shoulders. Arnica ointment is excellent for muscle cramps or spasms, as is eucalyptus oil and a compress of apple cider vinegar. Uranus is involved with the processes of oxygenation, so this placement can indicate an asthmatic tendency. Asthma responds well to acupuncture as well as to fenugreek tea and aloe vera. Eating lentils is also helpful. You are also subject to dry coughs. Wild cherry extract is good for coughs. Slippery elm is excellent for chest complaints. Gemini has general rulership over all the tubes in the body, so you can experience spasmodic constriction of one of the tubes of the body as well as muscular tics and twitches. A lack of vitamin E, magnesium, and vitamin B6 can lead to spastic conditions. The combination of Uranus and Gemini can indicate that you are high-strung, with a potential for nervous disorders. Chamomile tea and clove tea help quiet the nerves.

Uranus in Cancer

You are prone to a nervous stomach, with an uneven assimilation of food. You tend to have your own daily rhythm and may eat at odd hours, which can further contribute to poor assimilation of vitamins and minerals and contribute to stomach disorders. You are prone to spasmodic conditions of the stomach and stomach cramps and may become nauseous or vomit when under stress. You vary between an overacid and overalkaline stomach. Lettuce, carrots, and celery help promote alkalinity, which is considered conducive to good health. Chamomile tea soothes the stomach, as does cold sage tea. Both ginger and peppermint teas aid nausea.

Uranus in Leo

This placement is indicative of spasms in the back and the possibility of heart palpitations. There is a tendency toward arrhythmia. Your back can go out suddenly, especially when you are under stress or when bending over. You need to learn proper ways of bending and standing up and should avoid straining your back by trying to lift objects that are too heavy. There can be heart palpitations caused by a dysfunction of the thyroid gland. Lemon juice has a sedative action and can help nervous palpitations of the heart. Kelp is an aid to the thyroid, as are foods high in iodine, such as Swiss chard, watercress, broccoli, mushrooms, spinach, red cabbage, and potato skins. You are prone to valvular heart disease. If you suspect you have a heart disorder, you need to see your physician as soon as possible. You benefit from regular checkups with your doctor.

Uranus in Virgo

This placement can indicate an erratic pancreas. You can be prone to sugar-related problems such as diabetes or hypoglycemia. Eating too many rich, fatty foods puts a strain on the pancreas. Too much refined sugar in your diet can also cause havoc with the pancreas. The pancreas functions best when raw foods are eaten. With Virgo's association with the bowels, there can be cramping or diarrhea when nervous. Freshly grated nutmeg added to an herbal tea aids diarrhea. Chamomile and clove tea aid nervousness. You are prone to intestinal cramps and diseases such as colitis and Crohn's disease. Chlorophyll concentration added to water aids the bowels. Liver function can be erratic at times. Good nutrition and including foods such as raw nuts and seeds in the diet aid the liver.

Uranus in Libra

There can be irregular functioning of the kidneys. You are prone to lumbago (lower back pain) and abnormal kidney function when under stress. Regular exercise, using vitamin C, and learning how to bend properly can help prevent lumbago. Corn silk tea and pear juice promote kidney action. There can be skin eruptions brought on by shock. Good nutrition and possibly avoiding refined sugar, alcohol, coffee, strong spices, and cow's milk promote healthy skin and help prevent skin disorders. You are also prone to circulatory disorders. Rosemary is an aid to sluggish circulation.

Uranus in Scorpio

This placement indicates problems with the colon, causing diarrhea or constipation when under stress. You may have a spastic colon or other problems relating to the colon such as irritable bowel syndrome or colitis. Adding more fiber to the diet can promote colon health. Prunes, figs, and raw spinach salad can also help. During any flare-up, you need to eat easy-to-digest foods such as rice, sweet potatoes, steamed vegetables, and bananas. There can be bladder spasms or other bladder disorders. Lemon juice drinks are an aid to the bladder. In females, the monthly cycle may be irregular. Eating grated carrots that have been dried helps regulate menstruation.

Uranus in Sagittarius

You may be prone to overeating foods high in fat, which puts a strain on the liver. There can be accidents in sports activities and injuries to the hips and thighs, which need to be protected during vigorous activity. There can be cramps in the hips and thighs and a potential toward sciatica. Garlic and iodine are helpful against sciatica. Also helpful are eating potassium-rich foods such as bananas, oranges, and potatoes. You are also subject to blood disorders from eating an unhealthy diet. Onions and garlic are blood purifiers and aid circulation.

Uranus in Capricorn

There can be a problem in gallbladder action, which in turn causes problems with the function of the liver. Carrot, beet, and cucumber juice cleanse the gallbladder. There can be skin eruptions caused by stress or shock. Good nutrition and possibly avoiding refined sugar, alcohol, coffee, strong spices, and cow's milk promote healthy skin and help prevent skin disorders. There can be pain or cramping in your knees. Marjoram, plantain, comfrey,[14] and apple cider vinegar can all be used in a compress for swollen or painful knees. You are also prone to high cholesterol levels. Supplements such as acidophilus, activated charcoal, and calcium can help lower cholesterol levels.

Uranus in Aquarius

This placement aids your blood and circulation and facilitates good processes of oxygenation in the body. However, you are prone to nervous disorders and have a tendency to overreact emotionally, which can lead, in extreme cases, to hysteria. You benefit from the use of calming herbs such as bergamot and skullcap. Your lower legs and ankles are subject to cramping and accidents. Arnica ointment is excellent for muscle cramps or spasms, as is eucalyptus oil and a compress of apple cider vinegar.

Uranus in Pisces

You are prone to disorders of the feet such as spasm or cramping as well as excess perspiration. The feet can become swollen, and you are prone to corns and bunions. Acupressure can help alleviate foot pain. Massaging the soles also helps the feet. Tea tree oil and aloe vera gel soothe the feet. You may be diagnosed with a weird or unusual ailment, and you may also experience nervous disorders. Chamomile and clove tea aid nervousness.

Neptune in the Signs

The sign tenanted by Neptune can indicate a part of the body that has a lack of tone. It can be flabby or weak and needs to be nourished and stimulated. It is similar to the sign placement of Saturn in that it is considered a weak point in the body, where illness can develop. The sign placements of Saturn and Neptune can and should be read interchangeably. By sign placement, they tend to be the weakest points in the body. Neptune is, of course, a generational planet due to its slow motion, so the sign placement is not as important as the planetary aspects it makes. However, it should not be ignored if you are trying to build up your body. It behooves you to strengthen any weak part of your body to improve overall health. For more help, see Appendix A: Nutritional Guidance to Nourish Weak Areas of the Body.

Neptune in Aries

This placement can indicate weakened adrenal function and lowered immunity. There is susceptibility to infection and prolonged healing time. The adrenals benefit from pantothenic acid. Juices containing carrots, garlic, black currants, oranges, beets, green peppers, or watercress help build the immune system. There can be a weakness in the head area and poor teeth and gums. You may get infections in the mouth such as trench mouth. Goldenseal and myrrh are excellent for infections in the mouth. Goldenseal is also useful for the gums. Herbs such as sage or fenugreek can be used for a sore throat. You can also be prone to eye disorders such as conjunctivitis. Cucumber slices placed over the eyelids help with pink eye and eyestrain. Simple eye inflammation can be helped by eyebright tea. Serious eye disorders should be treated by a doctor.

Neptune in Taurus

This placement can indicate a weakness in the throat, neck, and thyroid areas. Vitamin E and iodine as well as iodized salt aid the thyroid. You would benefit from neck exercises to build up your neck muscles. You may be prone to throat infections or eruptions on the neck such as boils. Aloe vera gel and blackberry leaf tea can be used as topical applications for skin eruptions. Herbs such as sage or fenugreek can be used for a sore throat. The tonsils can become infected and may need to be removed. Tonsils benefit from gargling with a chlorophyll liquid concentrate.

Neptune in Gemini

This placement can indicate weak lungs and flabby arms and shoulders. You would probably be helped by lifting weights to build up your upper body. There is a weakness in the respiratory system and possible breathing disorders such as asthma or more serious disorders such as tuberculosis, pleurisy, or emphysema. Vitamin B6, vitamin C, vitamin A, and zinc can help prevent respiratory disorders. Asthma responds well to acupuncture. Garlic is helpful in lung disorders, as is wintergreen tea before retiring. Flaxseed tea, thyme, and comfrey[15] also aid the lungs.

Neptune in Cancer

This placement indicates poor digestion and the potential for conditions in the body such as candida, a yeast-like condition. This condition can be improved by avoiding products containing yeast, refined sugars, vinegars, mushrooms, aged cheese, dried fruits, and fruit juices. There may not be enough friendly bacteria in the stomach. This can be helped by adding yogurt to your diet. Women with this placement may have breast disease or a weakness in the womb area. Raspberry leaf tea is a tonic for women. In both sexes, the stomach tends toward flabbiness, which can be helped by exercises that strengthen the stomach muscles. You also benefit from upper body exercises to strengthen the chest, another weak area.

Neptune in Leo

You have a weak back, which can be strengthened by exercise. You need to use proper techniques for lifting heavy objects to avoid putting your back out. There is a weakness in the spinal area and a need to keep the spine and back supple. Adequate calcium in the diet is necessary to prevent back problems. A healthy spine needs calcium, magnesium, silicon, and vitamin B12. There can also be weakened heart action, prompting a need for cardiovascular exercises to build up the heart. Lecithin can be helpful for the heart. Borage strengthens the heart. Manganese helps protect the inside lining of the heart. Heavy coffee drinking may contribute to heart disease. It can be beneficial to eat more raw nuts and seeds for protein and less cheese and meat.

Neptune in Virgo

This placement can indicate a weak pancreas, causing blood sugar problems such as diabetes or misdiagnosed hypoglycemia. There can be mental confusion due to blood sugar problems. Eating too many rich, fatty foods puts a strain on the pancreas. Too much refined sugar in your diet can also cause havoc with the pancreas. There is a need to build up the enzyme action in the pancreas through the consumption of raw food. The bowels can be a weak area and require whole grains, fruits, and vegetables for proper elimination. Liver function can be sluggish. Dandelion root makes an excellent stimulant for the liver.

Neptune in Libra

This placement can indicate weak or sluggish kidney function or poor filtering of urine from the body, causing anemia and potential problems with the spleen. Toxins caused by a bad reaction to a drug can adversely affect your kidneys, and there is a need for pure food and water. Corn silk tea and pear juice promote kidney action. The electrolyte balance in the body can be off. Eye problems may be due to poor kidney function. Be careful of ingesting too much hard water, as this can adversely affect the kidneys. There can be an acid/alkaline imbalance in the body and a sodium imbalance. Alfalfa helps promote a healthy balance in the body. You should stay closer to an alkaline diet by eating foods such as berries, fresh vegetables, and milk products.

Neptune in Scorpio

You may have a weakness in the eliminative and reproductive organs. There can be poor peristalsis, causing problems with diarrhea or constipation. There is a need to add fiber to the diet to aid bowel function. There is the danger of infection in the reproductive system such as infections like vaginitis in females or a prostate infection in males. Women with this placement can use a calendula ointment, avoid yeast products, and eat more yogurt. Foods high in zinc such as pumpkin seeds and sunflower seeds aid the prostate. Both sexes are vulnerable to venereal diseases and need to practice safe sex. With reflex action to the throat, ruled by Taurus, the opposite sign, there can be throat problems or a hypothyroid condition. Vitamin E and iodine as well as iodized salt aid the thyroid. Herbs such as sage or fenugreek can be used for the throat.

Neptune in Sagittarius

There is a weakness in the area of the hips and thighs. There is the danger of hip injury through falling. Use care when walking on wet or icy sidewalks. There could also be ulcers on the hips. With reflex action to Gemini, the opposite sign, there can be lung infection and shallow breathing. You can benefit from diaphragmatic exercises, which aid the lungs. Flaxseed tea, thyme, and comfrey[16] nourish the lungs. There can be locomotor disorders due to a lack of tone in the hips and thighs. Exercises that strengthen the hips and thighs are beneficial.

Neptune in Capricorn

Your knees can be weak and need to be strengthened by exercise. You may experience swelling in this area. Marjoram, plantain, comfrey,[17] and apple cider vinegar can all be used in a compress for swollen knees. You are prone to skin infections that seep as well as a difficulty in healing. Skin conditions can be helped by the mineral qualities of cucumber and the healing qualities of aloe vera. There can be a weakness in the bones, leading to brittle bones. Juices containing carrots, garlic, black currants, oranges, beets, green peppers, or watercress help build the immune system and ability to heal. You can also benefit from dairy products such as yogurt, kefir, and buttermilk, as well as foods high in minerals such as sea vegetables, whole grains, and cabbage.

Neptune in Aquarius

You may be prone to nervous disorders. You benefit from calming herbs such as bergamot and skullcap to aid the nerves and lemon balm for relaxation and sleep. Calcium and magnesium are helpful in preventing nerve-related ailments. The circulation can be weak, and there can be weakened heart action. Onions and garlic are blood purifiers and aid circulation. You may be prone to infectious heart ailments such as endocarditis. If you suspect you have a heart ailment, you need to see your doctor immediately. Garlic and onions also aid the heart. Hawthorn is a heart tonic. There can be disorders due to your strong psychic sensitivity. You need to practice psychic self-defense.

Neptune in Pisces

There can be lowered immune function, creating a need to build up the immune system through both exercise and nutrition. Foods containing vitamins A, B, and C and zinc aid the immune system. Juices made from carrots, beets, lemons, oranges, green pepper, watercress, and parsley strengthen the immune system. There can be a water imbalance, resulting in edema. Grapes and celery are useful for edema, as is corn silk tea. The feet are weak, and you are prone to disorders such as athlete's foot and flat feet. Tea tree oil can be used for athlete's foot. Flat feet benefit from shoes with good support. You can be prone to unusual ailments and can be oversensitive to drugs. You may require a smaller dosage of a prescription.

Pluto in the Signs

It takes Pluto 284 years to go through each sign of the zodiac. Its effects in a sign appear to be entirely generational and too nonspecific for inclusion. Pluto should be examined as to its house position and aspects. See chapter 6 for a description of Pluto in the houses. See chapter 5 for a description of aspects involving Pluto.

---

1. Comfrey is best used externally as an ointment or as tincture drops in water made into a compress. Do not ingest, as some studies suggest that comfrey is carcinogenic in large doses.

2–17. Ibid.

5
The Aspects in Medical Astrology

Your birth chart is composed of planetary combinations, or aspects, that give you information about your health habits, nutritional needs, and factors that may affect health. Combinations of aspects with a similar theme can point to the potential for a specific disease or bodily weakness. The aspects in your chart are interpreted by beginning with the aspects your Sun makes to the other planets in your chart, followed by aspects made by the Moon, Mercury, Venus, Mars, Jupiter, Saturn, Uranus, Neptune, and Pluto. Also included are the aspects made to your Ascendant. (See "The Ascendant and the First House" in chapter 7.)

In general, the aspects are divided into what are known as hard or stressful aspects and soft or harmonious aspects. The major hard aspects used to interpret your chart are the square and opposition. The square aspect consists of planets in a 90° relationship to each other. Astrologers use orbs of allowable distance to determine the angular relationship between planets. Therefore, if an orb of 6° is used for a square, the allowable distance for two planets in a square aspect would be from 84° to 96° apart. The opposition aspect is 180°. The major soft aspects used to interpret your chart are the sextile and the trine. The sextile aspect is 60° and the trine is 120°. The conjunction is a major aspect consisting of two or more planets next to each other, and the meaning is colored by the nature of the planets involved, so it can be considered a hard or soft aspect.

It is important to remember that the following definitions of the major aspects in the birth chart are read strictly as planet to planet and do not take into account the rest of the aspects in your chart or the planets in the signs and houses. Therefore, you should use this information as a guide to the possibilities in your chart, which are modified, for better or worse, by the rest of your birth chart. It takes more than one planetary aspect in a chart to determine a condition. Use this information to guide you, but when you need more help, see a professional astrologer. For a summary of how each planet functions in medical astrology, see chapter 3. For additional information, see Appendix A: Nutritional Guidance to Nourish Weak Areas of the Body.

Sun Aspects

Sun Conjunct Moon

You may have energy problems and the potential for feverish or inflammatory complaints. Your energy fluctuates with your moods. You need to learn how to conserve your energy. There can be periods of emotional imbalance and a lack of objectivity. There is a strong identification between the feelings and the ego and a one-sidedness to the personality.

Sun Sextile/Trine Moon

This aspect aids emotional balance and vitality. Your inner and outer needs are in balance, and there is the ability to overcome fatigue and resist disease. You have a good sense of your body's natural rhythms and are able to conserve bodily energies. Psychological and physical health benefit from this aspect. Your constitution is strong and robust, and your body fluids are in balance. Eyesight tends to be equal in both eyes.

Sun Square/Opposition Moon

Your vitality is uneven and can depend on your emotional state. You have a tendency toward constitutional and functional disorders. You can be changeable and moody due to a conflict between the emotions and the will, leading to emotional highs and lows. When ill, you are susceptible to feverish or inflammatory complaints and a fluid imbalance in the body. There can be unequal sight in your eyes. You benefit from regular eye exams. Your system can be affected by cold, which can increase your susceptibility to colds and the flu. You benefit from increased fluids in the diet. You will find that your health improves with age. Nutritionally, you may have a deficiency of vitamin A, iodine, magnesium, and potassium.

Sun Conjunct Mercury

A conjunction is the only major aspect possible between the Sun and Mercury. This is because the Sun and Mercury can never be more than 28° apart. This aspect affects the nervous system and can indicate a tendency to be high-strung, anxious, and nervous. In extreme cases, one can experience mental disorders. There can be respiratory disorders and a hormonal imbalance. You need to learn to be more objective. You can benefit from eating foods containing thiamine and magnesium, such as green leafy vegetables and fruits and nuts.

Sun Conjunct Venus

You are friendly and warm, with a tendency toward self-indulgence. You have a slight propensity toward acidosis in the body, which can be helped by alfalfa, either as a tea or in tablet form. You may have a tendency toward excessive sugar consumption. A diet high in sugar can rob the body of needed nutrients and may play a role in such diseases as diabetes and hypoglycemia. A potential for impaired renal function can upset the acid/alkaline metabolism in the body. You may have a lack of body tone due to an aversion to exercise.

Sun Semisquare Venus

Based on the distance between the Sun and Venus, Venus can never be more than 48° from the Sun. Therefore, the only hard aspect between the two is called the semisquare. This aspect is 45°, or one-half of a square, which is 90°. There can be an acid/alkaline imbalance within the body. You may experience health problems due to excess. There is a need to curb your desire for sweets. Since Venus rules the venous circulation of the body, a hard aspect between the Sun and Venus can contribute to circulatory disorders. The equilibrium of the body is also altered with this aspect, leading to an imbalance of bodily energies. There can be poor functioning of the thyroid and other glandular disorders. You are prone to sore throats. This aspect also indicates a lack of vitamin E and vitamin A and a potential niacin deficiency.

Sun Conjunct Mars

Any aspect between the Sun and Mars is considered beneficial, as it aids in resistance to disease and gives the ability to fight infection. You have a strong constitution and much vitality. When ill, you have a feverish or inflammatory response, which helps burn off toxins in the body. You do have a tendency toward rash action and impulsiveness, which can lead to accidents. You need to learn how to pace yourself, as you have a tendency to work until physically exhausted, which puts too great a strain on the body.

Sun Sextile/Trine Mars

This is an aspect of good health, vitality, and longevity. The constitution is strong, and there is resistance to disease and healthy blood. You have a good metabolism, which aids in the utilization of food intake. The blood contains sufficient oxygen and iron. Your ego is strong, and you are energetic. You have a passion for life and are energized by hard work. You prefer to be active and can find a release from stress in sports and exercise. This aspect gives you the ability to fight disease, usually through fever or infection. You may be slightly acidic, which can upset the acid/alkaline balance in the body. Taking alfalfa as a tea or in tablet form can help restore the balance.

Sun Square/Opposition Mars

This aspect confers vitality, energy, and a fast metabolism, but your tendency toward hastiness or impulsiveness makes you accident-prone. This runs the gamut from scrapes and falls to burns or accidents from sharp instruments. A penchant to push yourself too hard can lead to sickness from overwork, muscle injury, and heart strain. There can be a rapid pulse. Cardiovascular disease can result from high blood pressure—this aspect is a factor in heart disease. The Sun in stressful aspect to Mars gives a feverish or inflammatory response to disease, which tends to be acute. The stomach can be sensitive and prone to acidosis, so you should watch your intake of spicy foods and high-acid foods such as meat, soft drinks, and white pasta. Since you have a fast metabolism, you do best eating frequent, small meals.

Sun Conjunct Jupiter

This aspect combines the best and worst of Sun-Jupiter, as it inclines toward immoderation. On the one hand, there can be vitality, endurance, and resistance to disease. You have an optimistic nature and healthy emotions, which are aids to good health. But a healthy appetite can put too much strain on the liver, leading to toxemia. There can be a difficulty in fat assimilation. You benefit from practicing moderation in food and drink.

Sun Sextile/Trine Jupiter

This aspect is an aid to good health and longevity. Your optimistic attitude promotes good health. There is endurance, vitality, and resistance to disease. There is healthy blood, and liver function is aided. A harmonious Sun-Jupiter aspect helps with the restoration of health after illness.

Sun Square/Opposition Jupiter

This aspect gives you vitality and energy, but you have a tendency toward excess in food and drink and a need for moderation. The appetite can be large, leading to weight gain and obesity. A life of excess can lead to a breakdown of health in the later years. Overindulgence in alcohol or protein-rich food can lead to increased levels of uric acid, a symptom of gout. You are susceptible to stroke. You may also have a difficulty in fat assimilation and may have trouble digesting foods high in fat. You need to be careful in the use of cooking oil, and should only use oils of the finest quality.

Blood cholesterol levels may be higher than normal and should be checked regularly by a doctor. You have a tendency toward disorders of the blood, leading to toxemia. Circulation can be sluggish, and there is the potential for high blood pressure. With a potential stress on the liver, eating apples, carrots, and zucchini can be beneficial to liver function. Lecithin flushes fat out of the liver and increases liver function. The liver also benefits from vitamin A, chlorine, sulphur, and iodine.

Sun Conjunct Saturn

You have endurance and strength. Your natural tendency toward moderation is an aid to good health and longevity, as you tend to choose foods that are good for you. You may have a weakness in the bones and teeth, with a tendency toward poor circulation. Exercise is needed to keep the joints and muscles limber and for improved cardiovascular action. An overly rigid nature can contribute to stiff joints and energy blocks. You benefit from yoga-type exercises and body massage.

Sun Sextile/Trine Saturn

The constitution is strong, with endurance and a good body structure. There is the ability to withstand disease. This aspect gives a disciplined and sensible nature, which helps prevent excess in the diet and also helps prevent accidents. You have good common sense, which helps you choose foods that are good for you, such as raw foods, which help extend life. You have healthy bones and teeth.

Sun Square/Opposition Saturn

You can have energy problems and decreased resistance to disease with a hard aspect between the Sun and Saturn. Disease can be hereditary, and there is the potential for chronic disease, depletion of energy, and lowered vitality. The appetite can be poor, and you have a tendency toward alkalinity. Your metabolism is slow, causing food to take longer to be digested. You should avoid heavy foods, such as too much meat and potatoes, which slow digestion. Eating periodic, large meals can be detrimental to your health, as you do better with small, frequent meals.

Sun-Saturn combinations can indicate bone conditions, poor circulation, and dental troubles. There is a tendency toward illnesses arising from cold or neglect. You are also prone to conditions such as rheumatism, arthritis, and arteriosclerosis as well as calcification caused by an accumulation of mineral deposits in the body tissues or structures. The spine can be weak, and there can be locomotor problems. You may have a deficiency of vitamins A, C, and D, and may require more calcium. You benefit from techniques that release blocked energy and tension, such as chiropractic adjustment or deep body massage.

Sun Conjunct Uranus

This combination of Sun and Uranus indicates that you are a nervous, erratic type, with a strong, individualistic nature. You can become easily excited or even hysterical. The herb rosemary helps prevent hysterical outbursts. Your strong need to assert your individuality can put a strain on the nervous system, contributing to nervous or circulatory disorders. You should use care to avoid accidents around electrical equipment. There can be diseases resulting in incoordination.

Sun Sextile/Trine Uranus

You have a high energy level and good circulation. Your mind is alert and original. You may be into the latest health fad, but as you are scientifically oriented, you are able to distinguish between quackery and what is useful. Breathing exercises and the avoidance of polluted air aid your health. Outdoor exercise helps you reduce stress.

Sun Square/Opposition Uranus

You are high-strung, with an uneven energy level. You can be prone to high blood pressure, which is relieved by simple living, fresh air, and rest. You may experience nervous disorders, spasm conditions, cold sweats, circulatory problems, and heart palpitations. You benefit from calming foods such as celery, turkey, bananas, figs, chamomile tea, and valerian tea. You are prone to rare ailments. You are susceptible to changes in barometric pressure, which can lead to nervousness or moodiness. You need to be careful around electrical appliances, as there can be accidents involving electricity. There can be disorders of the blood, causing anemia. Foods high in iron, such as apples, beets, apricots, broccoli, blueberries, raisins, spinach, whole wheat, almonds, dates, and wheat germ, help prevent anemia.

Sun Conjunct Neptune

You are idealistic and insightful but have a delicate body. Your desire to serve others can cause an energy drain, either mentally or physically, unless you put limits on your time. Your supersensitivity makes it difficult for you to ward off negative influences around you—these run the gamut from picking up negative emotions from persons in your environment to a susceptibility to toxins in the air. You need to practice psychic self-defense by putting up an invisible wall around yourself for self-protection. You tend toward allergies or lowered resistance, which causes you to catch colds and flus. There is a need to pay attention to your diet and include fresh fruits and vegetables on a daily basis. You need to get adequate rest and sleep to aid your immune system.

Sun Sextile/Trine Neptune

This aspect confers a favorable influence. It is sometimes considered an angelic benediction and could result in a spiritual healing. You, yourself, may have healing ability. You could benefit from outdoor exercise and water therapies. You have great inspiration and the ability to use common sense and adopt natural health measures, which contribute to good health.

Sun Square/Opposition Neptune

This aspect can weaken the health and cause vitality problems. You have a high degree of physical sensitivity, causing you to experience periodic declines. There can be psychic disorders, weakened heart action, and prolonged healing time. Immunity can be low, and there is a propensity toward anemia or problems with iron assimilation. Engaging in some form of exercise can increase vitality and add body tone. Engaging in artistic activities involving music or the arts can also help restore vitality.

There can be body toxicity. You may be prone to infections, continual colds, flus, and swollen lymph glands. Sun-Neptune contacts can indicate the potential for misdiagnosis, and you should get a second opinion on any serious health matter. There can be poor assimilation of vitamins and minerals. There is a potential for edema, which can be caused by a sodium/potassium imbalance.

You need to build up your immune system. Cutting down on refined products and products containing white flour, white sugar, and white rice is a first step. The immune system is also aided by increased protein, supplements such as acidophilus, vitamin A, vitamin C, zinc, and magnesium, and herbs such as thyme, rosemary, and garlic.

You are most likely drug-sensitive and may require only half the dosage prescribed. You are easily addicted to substances such as drugs or alcohol, and you can become overly dependent on stimulants such as coffee and cigarettes. You may be allergic to synthetic fibers or animal fur and be prone to food allergies, especially to seafood. You are also highly sensitive to preservatives and coloring agents used to prepare foods. You should wash your fruits and vegetables carefully, as you can also have an allergic reaction to insecticides used in growing fruits and vegetables. If possible, you should eat only organic fruits and vegetables. You may also be allergic to everyday household cleaning agents, especially cleaning sprays containing harsh chemicals. Skin irritation could be caused by detergents and fabric softeners. It is important to have your eyes checked once or twice a year, as there can be vision problems with this aspect.

Sun Conjunct Pluto

You are intense and observant and have a clear understanding of the use of energy. You have good recuperative powers and the ability to regenerate yourself and others. You have a strong constitution, with the ability to resist disease. However, you don't always recognize the limits of your body and can push yourself to extremes, which can lead to a breakdown in health in your later years. You need to learn to pace yourself.

Sun Sextile/Trine Pluto

You have strong recuperative powers, with the ability to resist disease. You are able to continually transform your body and mind, leading to improved health. There is a toughness to the constitution and good endurance. You are able to overcome most threats to health.

Sun Square/Opposition Pluto

You are tough and resilient, with a sound constitution. You have a powerful personality and much drive but tend to push yourself to the limits of your body's endurance, causing a breakdown in health and a fluctuating recuperative ability. You are prone to infection, stress-related illnesses, swellings, and abscesses. Outdoor exercise helps you reduce stress. Hard Sun-Pluto aspects are also associated with drastic health measures.

Moon Aspects

Moon Conjunct Mercury

It can be difficult for you to separate your emotions from your thinking processes, as they are so intertwined. This lack of objectivity can lead to anxiety and worry. Negative thinking can depress the immune system and also lead to depression. A constant need to be busy can put a strain on the nervous system and cause difficulties in sleeping. There is a need for you to cultivate tranquility.

Moon Sextile/Trine Mercury

You have a good memory and a sound nervous system, and tend to be sensible and reliable. You practice good hygiene and know the value of a healthy diet in resisting disease. You can pace yourself and know how to utilize your energy.

Moon Square/Opposition Mercury

You are sensitive to outside stimuli, tend to be nervous, and have a tendency to worry too much. You may be prone to respiratory or allergic disorders such as hay fever or asthma. You are easily upset and can appear high-strung and neurotic. Your inability to relax puts a lot of stress on your nervous system. You may have insomnia. You may also have difficulty concentrating, leading to memory problems or absent-mindedness. There can be too much worry over health and a need to cultivate positive thinking. You can benefit from using relaxation techniques such as meditation or yoga or allowing yourself quiet times to read and relax.

Moon Conjunct Venus

You are easygoing, with a positive mental outlook. You enjoy the good things in life, especially food and drink. In fact, you may ignore healthy foods if they don't appeal to your palate in favor of non-nutritious, empty-calorie foods. Illness can be due to overindulgence. A craving for sweets can lead to dental problems or obesity. Laziness can lead to flabbiness, as it can be difficult for you to engage in a regular physical exercise regimen. Joining a health club or engaging in activities such as yoga or walking would add tone to your body.

Moon Sextile/Trine Venus

You are charming and friendly and are usually emotionally content. Your positive attitude is an aid to good health. This aspect strengthens the constitution, digestive processes, and circulation of the body. It is an aid to women, as it usually indicates easy conception.

Moon Square/Opposition Venus

You are prone to health disorders caused by excess. This can be due to a sweet tooth or just overindulgence in foods that provide little nutrition. A difficulty in achieving emotional satisfaction can lead to overeating, which can lead to digestive disturbances or a general imbalance in the body. Women with this aspect can be prone to female problems such as PMS, swollen breasts, or a water imbalance in the body. Red raspberry leaf is an excellent herb for women with these problems. There can be altered bodily rhythms and hormonal problems. There can also be poor body tone due to a lack of exercise.

Moon Conjunct Mars

Your emotions run high, and there can be an urgency to the personality. You can be hyper and impatient, which puts a strain on your nervous system, and your impatience and irritability can lead to stomach upsets that range from an acid stomach to an ulcer. You need to learn relaxation techniques and to keep your anger under control. Stimulants such as coffee and colas and foods such as aged cheese and soy sauce can have a strong effect on you, possibly in the form of headaches. Herbal teas such as chamomile or valerian could have a soothing effect on your body.

Moon Sextile/Trine Mars

You are endowed with tremendous vitality and a strong constitution. You are able to surmount most threats to health. Drugs or alcohol can have a negative effect on your system and should be used in moderation. Females born with harmonious Moon-Mars aspects have healthy reproductive systems and are usually able to avoid female complaints like PMS or the negative effects of menopause.

Moon Square/Opposition Mars

Though you have tremendous vitality and a strong sense of self, your overaggressive and impatient attitude can lead to a variety of health problems. These can be minor, such as digestive upsets, nausea, or skin eruptions, or more serious conditions, such as high blood pressure or ulcers. You are also prone to accidents, especially with sharp objects or hot water. You have a tendency to overreact emotionally to trivial matters, making yourself and others nervous and ill at ease. Females born with this aspect are subject to menstrual irregularities and a difficult pregnancy, with the potential for miscarriage.

You need to learn how to deal with anger in a more constructive way and would benefit from anger-management therapy. Highly spiced foods can have an adverse effect on your stomach. You are prone to inflammatory disorders and would benefit from calming foods such as celery, bananas, turkey, and figs.

Moon Conjunct Jupiter

This aspect gives optimism and exuberance, which are beneficial to health. There is much vitality. You may have a sweet tooth or a craving for foods high in fat, which can be a deterrent to good health and can lead to obesity. There can be digestive problems involving the gallbladder and liver. You may have difficulty digesting fried, fatty, and oily foods, so your consumption of these should be kept to a minimum. You are also prone to blood disorders. Toxins from overindulgence of food, especially alcohol, can put a strain on the liver. Liver ailments could be helped by supplementing your diet with lecithin and aloe vera and including foods such as apples, carrots, zucchini, goat's milk, and raw and unsalted nuts and seeds.

Moon Sextile/Trine Jupiter

Your generous and optimistic attitude is an aid to good health. You are able to heal yourself and others with your magnetism and vitality. You have good common sense, which helps you avoid excess in your diet, and you tend toward a healthy lifestyle. Women with this aspect are usually able to conceive and have a healthy pregnancy.

Moon Square/Opposition Jupiter

You are optimistic and generous but can be highly emotional, with a tendency toward extravagance, especially in eating and drinking. Overindulgence in fatty, fried, or oily foods puts a strain on the liver, causes a difficulty in fat assimilation, and contributes to body toxicity. Excessive alcohol intake can lead to cirrhosis of the liver. There can be digestive problems involving the gallbladder and liver. You may contract blood disorders and eruptive diseases, boils, and pimples from blood impurities. Red clover tea is a blood purifier. There can also be excess uric acid production in the body, which can lead to gout. Your hips and thighs are also vulnerable parts of your body. Females with this aspect may experience tenderness of the breasts or fluid retention.

Moon Conjunct Saturn

You have endurance and a strong constitution. You use good common sense combined with good health habits that are conducive to preventing disease and aiding longevity. There can be some tendency toward rigidity, leading to conditions such as stiff joints or arthritis. The bones and teeth are also vulnerable. A tendency toward somberness can be counteracted by engaging in activities that you enjoy.

Moon Sextile/Trine Saturn

You are sensible and conscientious, with the discipline to do what is necessary for good health. You are able to adopt good health habits that are conducive to old age. You have a strong constitution, with much endurance. You have willpower and stamina and tend toward moderation, which helps keeps the bodily energies balanced. You tend to choose foods that are good for you.

Moon Square/Opposition Saturn

You may have difficulty expressing yourself due to a lack of self-esteem. On a psychological level, there can be a fear of change, moodiness, a depressed attitude, and excessive worry over minor matters. This anxiety can manifest as digestive problems, stiff joints, poor circulation, and bladder disease. You have a tendency to retain fluids. There is a disturbance of the water balance in the body, which causes a lack of moisture in the mucous membranes of the body, leading to dryness. This can result in soreness or stiffness in various parts of the body. Eating fruits and vegetables with a high water content is helpful. These include melons and celery. You are vulnerable to respiratory disorders and conditions arising from the cold or poor nutrition. Women with this aspect are prone to female disorders such as breast cysts or fibroid tumors and may have a difficult pregnancy. Raspberry leaf tea is an excellent tonic for women.

Moon Conjunct Uranus

Your behavior is erratic and you tend to overact emotionally, putting a strain on your nervous system. You can be stubborn and willful. You can be high-strung and nervous. Though highly original and independent, you can appear moody and unpredictable to others. You may have sudden mood swings, and this combined with an erratic disposition can lead to stomach upsets of a spastic nature. A lack of vitamin B6 and magnesium can contribute to spastic conditions, which are also helped by vitamin E. You seek excitement and unique adventures but need to learn to relax and develop a more contemplative attitude.

Moon Sextile/Trine Uranus

You are exciting and original. You seek unique and unusual people to help you. You are always ready to try the latest diet fad. A desire for constant stimulation can put a strain on the nervous system. You may benefit from juices, fasts, the use of acupuncture or colonics, and eating more raw food.

Moon Square/Opposition Uranus

You are exciting and original and like to operate at high tension. This puts a strain on your nervous system, which can lead to a breakdown in health. You can be willful and overexcitable. At the extreme, people with this aspect could have a nervous breakdown. Normally, you can expect to have digestive upsets, disorders of blood pressure, or circulatory disorders. There can be conditions involving spasms, twitching, or some form of incoordination. There can be accidents involving electricity. Women with this aspect may experience ovulatory pain, menstrual irregularities, or miscarriage. You need to learn how to ground yourself and to allow yourself soothing periods of quiet and relaxation. Eating heavy foods can help ground you. These include root vegetables—carrots, potatoes, turnips, beets, and squash. You can also benefit by including whole grains, brown rice, nuts, oils, cheese, butter, garlic, onions, and spices such as ginger and curry in your diet. You may need more B-complex vitamins and magnesium.

Moon Conjunct Neptune

Though highly imaginative, intuitive, and sensitive, you have a tendency toward escapism in order to avoid the harsh realities of life. You are susceptible to suggestion and may have an addictive personality. This can take the form of drug or alcohol abuse, overeating, or even watching too much television. Healthwise, you may have strong food sensitivities that trigger allergic reactions, which can manifest as skin disorders, respiratory ailments, or stomach upset. There can also be allergies to shellfish. You would benefit from warm baths and using soothing body oils.

Moon Sextile/Trine Neptune

You are sensitive and intuitive, with much compassion for others. You may have healing ability. Your strong spiritual beliefs are an aid to good health, and there can also be a spiritual healing at some point in your life. You benefit from water therapies such as swimming and bathing, which have a soothing effect on your psyche. You do well on a diet of natural foods.

Moon Square/Opposition Neptune

You are oversensitive, can have difficulty accepting reality, and can be fearful, with fanciful imaginings. You tend toward a great deal of anxiety. This aspect can adversely affect mental health, and there is a strong need for grounding. Occasionally eating heavy foods, such as meat and potatoes, helps keep you grounded. Root vegetables such as carrots, turnips, beets, and squash are also grounding.

You are prone to allergies and may have food and environmental sensitivities. You can easily become addicted to substances such as drugs, alcohol, coffee, or junk food. Watching television is also an addictive escape. Illness can be misdiagnosed, and you can be oversensitive to prescription drugs, requiring only half the normal dosage. You may have unusual cravings, psychosomatic illnesses, and allergic reactions to seafood. There can be female disorders and a weakness in the female organs.

You have a tendency to retain water. You benefit from restricting salt intake and eating diuretic foods such as celery and watermelon. Foods should be as pure as possible. You can also be helped by taking cell salts and following a detoxification diet.

Moon Conjunct Pluto

You have tremendous vitality and energy, with the ability to positively transform your body. You are able to use psychological insight in solving your problems, and others turn to you for help and advice. A tendency toward extremes and obsessive-compulsive behavior strains the body, causing stomach upsets and other problems such as hypertension, constipation, or headaches. Channeling your emotions into a special project helps draw out negative emotions.

Moon Sextile/Trine Pluto

You are psychologically astute, with tremendous vitality and a strong constitution. This aspect strengthens the female functions as well as the reproductive and eliminative organs of the body for both sexes. You have the ability to regenerate yourself to improve health. Your therapeutic skills are an aid in helping others.

Moon Square/Opposition Pluto

You are a person of extremes who tends to see things in black and white. You are psychologically acute but mentally intense and inflexible to the point where there can be mental obsessions or disorders or body toxicity. Your extreme mood swings can be disconcerting to others in your presence. Women with this aspect are subject to fibroid tumors and menstrual irregularities. There is also the danger of miscarriage. This aspect can also indicate a blood disease, disturbance of the bowels, and surgery on the colon. Ginger is an excellent detoxifier for the body.

Mercury Aspects

Mercury Conjunct Venus

This aspect confers a quiet disposition and ease of expression. There can be laxity or a lazy attitude in regard to health or minor disorders due to excess. You may have occasional nervous irritation, as the sensory nerves are vulnerable.

Mercury Sextile Venus

Mercury and Venus are able to reach a sextile aspect of 60°, though they are unable to form a trine of 120° due to their distance from each other in the solar system. This aspect confers good cheer and a sound mental outlook. The nervous system is strengthened, and there is the ability to handle stress.

Mercury Semisquare Venus

On its own, this aspect may cause one to be lax in health habits or overindulge in sweets. There can be a weakness in the intestines or problems with the general health of the nervous system. This planetary pair refers to sensory nerves, so in combination with other difficult aspects to Mercury, there is a vulnerability in this area. There can also be glandular disorders. Ginseng helps as a glandular and body balancer.

Mercury Conjunct Mars

You have a sharp and quick mind and good reflexes. You tend to be impatient with others, causing yourself nervous tension. You like to keep busy and may not allow yourself enough rest. You have busy hands, which are subject to accidents such as a wrist injury or broken finger, and there can be damage to the tendons from repetitive motion leading to disorders such as carpel tunnel syndrome.

Mercury Sextile/Trine Mars

You have a sound nervous system and good coordination. Your mind is sharp, and your memory is good. You are resourceful when it comes to solving health problems and can usually find a quick cure. You enjoy exercise, especially muscle building, which gives you added stamina and endurance.

Mercury Square/Opposition Mars

You are a person who likes speed and excitement. You tend to eat too quickly or on the run, which can lead to an acid stomach or bowel irritation. You are subject to nervous disorders, nerve inflammation, joint inflammation, intestinal disturbances, and excess uric acid caused by eating too much protein or from alcohol indulgence. You have a tendency to overwork the mind and to exaggerate matters out of proportion. A difficulty in turning off the mind causes insomnia or headaches. You have a low pain threshold and can experience anxiety, especially before dental visits. There is the potential for increased nerve irritability, leading to problems with the motor nerves in the body. Chamomile tea and clove tea help soothe the nerves. There can be a tendency to contract diseases such as Bell's palsy.

Mercury Conjunct Jupiter

You are optimistic and cheerful, which is beneficial to good health. You have good common sense and a desire for a healthful lifestyle. Your tendency toward extravagance can contribute to overindulgence in food and drink. The intestines are vulnerable and there is the potential for bowel disorders.

Mercury Sextile/Trine Jupiter

Your cheerfulness and optimistic attitude are aids to good health. You use good common sense in diet and exercise, and you are knowledgeable about the latest medical breakthroughs. You tend toward traditional health therapies over alternative healing methods.

Mercury Square/Opposition Jupiter

You are hopeful and cheerful but have a tendency to overindulge in rich foods. This can put a strain on the liver and can cause a difficulty in fat assimilation. There can be bowel disorders and blood impurities. You are sensitive to large amounts of coffee, tea, or cola, which can irritate your nervous system and cause headaches or dizziness. Continued use of these substances can lead to diseases of the pancreas or to nervous disorders. When ill, you tend to ignore good advice, as you have a "know-it-all" attitude.

Mercury Conjunct Saturn

You are logical, organized, and dependable. You prefer to follow traditional methods of healing. You like to stick to the tried and true and may not allow enough variety in your diet. You do like to follow a specific daily health regimen, which is an aid to longevity. You can be a bit rigid and may contract disorders such as arthritis and joint pain.

Mercury Sextile/Trine Saturn

You have good common sense and tend to follow a health regimen geared toward keeping the mind and body strong. You have a healthy nervous system and a sound body structure. Your nerves are steady, giving you the ability to handle stress.

Mercury Square/Opposition Saturn

You have a tendency to be fearful and anxious and can become easily discouraged or depressed. An overly rigid disposition can lead to stiffness or pain in the joints, numbness in the hands and arms, or disorders such as arthritis. There can be nerve inhibition, numbness of nerves, and poor reflex action. This planetary combination is also involved in hearing disorders, respiratory disorders, and problems with the intestinal tract causing constipation and a lack of healthy bacterial flora in the body. There can be insufficient mucus secretion on the respiratory membranes. This aspect has been associated with speech and hearing problems such as stuttering, stammering, and dyslexia. There can be an increased need for vitamin B6.

Mercury Conjunct Uranus

Your have an active intellect, are curious and progressive, and like to keep up with the latest health trends. You can be high-strung, with a sensitive nervous system, which needs to be pampered by periods of low stimulus. You are very energetic but would gain more strength through exercise and building up your muscles instead of your tendency to run on nervous energy.

Mercury Sextile/Trine Uranus

You are insightful, progressive, and scientifically minded. You are open to new ideas and are not afraid to try an unusual health regimen if you think it will improve your health. Easily bored, you are one of the first to try the latest diet fad. Daily exercise helps channel your nervous energy.

Mercury Square/Opposition Uranus

You are highly energetic, with a fast metabolism. You would benefit from eating small, frequent meals instead of large ones, as this will help to restore the energy you so quickly use up. You tend to be high-strung and scattered, which can put a strain on your nervous system, leading to such conditions as headaches, spasms, or twitching. You may need more of the B vitamins, especially thiamine. Constant pressure and a difficulty in handling stress can put too much strain on your sensitive nerves and can lead to nerve irritation or, at worst, a nervous breakdown. You may be prone to worry and anxiety. You need daily exercise to help you deal with stress and to help channel your nervous energy.

Mercury Conjunct Neptune

You have a psychic sensitivity to outside stimuli and can pick up negative vibrations from your surroundings or be prone to environmental allergies. You are drug-sensitive and may require only half the usual dosage of a medication. You have a tendency toward worry and anxiety and can be irrational and dreamy. You benefit from grounding techniques such as gardening and eating more root vegetables.

Mercury Sextile/Trine Neptune

You are imaginative and visionary. When ill, you do well with guided imagery that helps you visualize a healthy body. Your strong spiritual nature gives you a sense of well-being and security, which is an aid to good health.

Mercury Square/Opposition Neptune

You can have a problem dealing with reality and prefer to live in a dream world. You tend to delude yourself and can be fearful and irrational. At worst, there can be a mental imbalance. Constant worry can have a deleterious effect on your health. There is danger through the use of substances such as drugs or alcohol, which you tend to abuse. Smoking adversely affects your lungs and nervous system. Your nerves are weak, which can contribute to such disorders as nerve paralysis, numbness, palsy, and a decreased ability to feel or sense. Vitamin B is important for nerve health. There can be eye problems such as squinting or cataracts.

Mercury Conjunct Pluto

You have a penetrating and resourceful mind. You have much psychological insight, which you use to help yourself and others. You can be mentally intense and obsessive. This obsessiveness can strain the body, leading to nerve irritation. You may have an imbalance of the B vitamins. There can be thyroid problems, respiratory disorders such as pneumonia, or a hormonal imbalance in the body.

Mercury Sextile/Trine Pluto

You have a sound nervous system, are psychologically acute, and are able to handle stress. You are interested in the latest scientific breakthroughs affecting health. You have much stamina and are able to resist infection. When ill, you use investigative skills before deciding on a course of action. You function well under pressure and do best when using your strong mental abilities.

Mercury Square/Opposition Pluto

You are a person with great mental intensity, but you have a tendency to be compulsive and obsessive. This can put a strain on the nervous system, leading to nerve irritation. A nervous disorder could also be linked to your thyroid. You are prone to respiratory disorders and infectious disorders such as viral pneumonia. You do not handle stress well and are prone to stress-related ailments such as hypertension and insomnia. You need to allow yourself periods of low stimulus and relaxation.

Venus Aspects

Venus Conjunct Mars

Your kidneys are vulnerable and prone to irritation. You are susceptible to skin irritation and throat disorders as well as problems with the venous circulation of the body. Your sensuality and sensuousness can lead to sexual excesses. There is a need to guard against sexually transmitted diseases such as herpes by practicing safe sex.

Venus Sextile/Trine Mars

You have abundant energy, healthy sexual urges, and good kidney action. The reproductive organs function well, and this aspect is an aid for any women desiring to become pregnant. It aids fertility in both sexes. Venus in harmonious aspect to Mars is also favorable for the venous circulation of the body.

Venus Square/Opposition Mars

You are very passionate, with strong sensual desires. In both sexes, there is the danger of diseases of the reproductive organs. There can be an acid/alkaline imbalance in the body and the potential for kidney infection. You may experience renal irritation or skin ailments caused by kidney dysfunction. Women with this configuration can have menstrual difficulties or ovarian or bladder infections. There can be problems with the venous circulation of the body, leading to such conditions as varicose veins or phlebitis. Sufficient vitamin E is essential for healthy veins.

Venus Conjunct Jupiter

You are sociable and optimistic. You love to have a good time, which can lead to health problems caused by excess. With Venus ruling sugar and Jupiter ruling fat, you have a tendency to indulge in foods high in both. There can be a lazy attitude toward health and a tendency to take your good health for granted. You need to exercise and follow a stricter health regimen.

Venus Sextile/Trine Jupiter

This is a positive aspect that gives optimism and healthy emotions. This aspect promotes longevity. There can be a slight tendency toward self-indulgence, especially in sugary products, and a need for more exercise.

Venus Square/Opposition Jupiter

You are friendly and sociable but can have a lazy attitude in regard to your health. There is a tendency toward excesses in eating, which can lead to weight gain and also strain the liver function, leading to a build-up of toxins in the body. You may benefit from a supervised fruit fast. There can be problems with the venous circulation of the body, leading to conditions such as varicose veins or phlebitis. Females with this aspect are prone to glandular malfunctions due to a hormonal imbalance. Men with this aspect tend to become overweight or have a lack of body tone due to a lack of exercise and overindulgence in sugary and fatty foods.

Venus Conjunct Saturn

You are serious and disciplined in mind and body. You are careful in your choice of foods and have strong willpower. The kidneys can be a weak area of the body, with the potential for kidney stones. The venous circulation of the body can be sluggish. There can be glandular malfunction, especially of the thyroid.

Venus Sextile/Trine Saturn

This aspect confers good health and promotes healthy kidney action. You know how to conserve energy and pace yourself. You use good common sense in the choice of foods, aiding longevity.

Venus Square/Opposition Saturn

Your kidneys are vulnerable and may not function up to par, leading to disorders such as kidney stones or kidney obstruction. There can be a suppression of urine. You have a tendency toward dry skin and are prone to skin disorders. Good nutrition and possibly avoiding refined sugar, alcohol, coffee, strong spices, and cow's milk promote healthy skin and help prevent skin disorders. You are also prone to circulatory disorders. Women may experience a malfunction in the secretion of female hormones. There can also be an acid/alkaline imbalance in the body and problems with the veins that involve venous elasticity. The throat is a sensitive area, and the thyroid can underfunction. The thyroid is helped by foods high in iodine, such as seaweed and dulse.

Venus Conjunct Uranus

You are exciting and scintillating, with a strong libido. You are easily bored and have a tendency to be high-strung. You can appear nervous and excitable. There is some tendency toward problems with the venous circulation in the body and the potential for heart palpitations.

Venus Sextile/Trine Uranus

You have a scintillating personality and a strong desire for emotional freedom. You enjoy a variety of foods, which is an aid to good health. This is a positive aspect that adds to feelings of well-being and aids the circulation of the body and kidney function.

Venus Square/Opposition Uranus

You are excitable and easily bored. You may have poor circulation, especially of the extremities. You may have episodes of spasmodic kidney pain, a heart murmur, or heart palpitations. You have a progressive attitude toward sex and need to guard against sexual excess.

Venus Conjunct Neptune

You are a dreamy and idealistic person. You are not always realistic and can ignore messages from your body. There can be a flabbiness or water imbalance in the tissues. You may have a hormonal imbalance. You have escapist tendencies and may tend to overuse drugs or alcohol. You may also be prone to allergies or weakened kidney action.

Venus Sextile/Trine Neptune

You are a dreamer, with much vision and inspiration. You are in tune with nature and do well on a natural diet. Delving into creative or spiritual activities brings you peace of mind, which is an aid to good health. You have natural healing abilities.

Venus Square/Opposition Neptune

You can be spacey, unrealistic, and neurotic. You can be hypersensitive to toxins in the air or other allergens such as food additives or preservatives. You may be drug-sensitive, requiring lower dosages than what is prescribed. You may have allergic reactions to some varieties of seafood. Your metabolism can be upset or out of balance. The sugar metabolism in your body can be out of whack. There is a tendency toward alcohol or drug abuse, which can lead to a breakdown in the body. Women may have a weakened glandular function, leading to a weakness in the female reproductive system. There can be flabbiness due to lack of exercise or a water imbalance in the body.

Venus Conjunct Pluto

You are intense and complicated, with a tendency toward deep feelings. You are prone to stress-related disorders. There can also be endocrine disorders, skin conditions or skin diseases, and infections of the reproductive organs for both males and females. The throat is vulnerable, and there is the potential for throat infections.

Venus Sextile/Trine Pluto

You are sensual and magnetic. You have a healthy attitude about love and sex. This aspect aids the endocrine system in the body and promotes healthy skin. It also promotes good kidney action.

Venus Square/Opposition Pluto

You have an intense nature, with an all-or-nothing approach to life. You may obsess to the point of neurosis. Your extremist tendencies can manifest as extremes in diet or exercise routines, which can aversely affect health. You are prone to skin growths such as acne and warts or fungus-like conditions. Women with this aspect may have excessive glandular secretions, which interfere with the female cycle. This aspect is associated with poor sugar metabolism in the body. You may have a chromium deficiency.

Mars Aspects

Mars Conjunct Jupiter

You are energetic and enthusiastic, with a desire to live an active life. You enjoy physical exercise or any physical activity that allows you to expend energy. You have healthy blood and a sound physical body, with a good metabolism and excellent muscular action. You have strong resistance to disease. With your abundance of energy and overexuberance, there can be injuries to the muscles or a tendency toward conditions such as sciatica. Garlic and iodine are helpful against sciatica.

Mars Sextile/Trine Jupiter

You have a healthy body, with much power and vitality. You are optimistic and have the ability to overcome and resist disease You have sufficient iron in the blood, which aids oxygenation. This aspect also aids liver function and indicates smooth muscle activity in the body.

Mars Square/Opposition Jupiter

You are generally optimistic, with much endurance and the ability to fight disease. Generally, you have a rich blood supply. You have a tendency toward exaggeration and overindulgence, which can lead to disorders caused by excess. You should avoid overly rich and fatty foods. There can be blood disorders, muscle injuries, and liver complaints. Liver ailments could be helped by supplementing your diet with lecithin and aloe vera and eating foods such as apples, carrots, zucchini, goat's milk, and raw and unsalted nuts and seeds. You are prone to sciatica and arthritis. Garlic and iodine are helpful against sciatica. You tend to push yourself too hard to the point of exhaustion and need to learn the limits of your body.

Mars Conjunct Saturn

You are disciplined and have much endurance. You have strong determination but can become obsessive and compulsive. This strains your body and can lead to muscular tension, stiff muscles, or joint inflammation. Physical exercise can help keep you limber. There is the danger of falls, bruises, dental problems, and blood ailments. You tend to run hot and cold both physically and emotionally, resulting in energy blocks, frustration, and indecision. You have to learn how to deal with anger. You prefer the traditional approach to solving health problems.

Mars Sextile/Trine Saturn

You have a sound body structure and the energy to accomplish difficult tasks. There is endurance and resistance to disease. You have strength in your bones and muscles. Your teeth and gums are healthy and benefit from fresh fruits and vegetables.

Mars Square/Opposition Saturn

You are prone to conditions affecting your body structure such as arthritis and rheumatism. You may have energy blocks and become easily frustrated. This aspect can adversely affect the joints, bones, and muscles of the body. Mars-Saturn combinations can indicate rigid muscles, joint inflammation, or problems with the tendons or cartilage. Therapies such as massage or movements such as yoga or dancing are beneficial. You are also vulnerable to injuries to the skin, falls, and bruises, and have the potential to develop gallstones. There can be bowel disorders, leading to constipation. There can be a tendency toward blood ailments, most likely anemia caused by poor iron absorption. Eating foods high in vitamin C is beneficial. It is important to see your dentist frequently, as there can be dental problems. Glandular disorders could manifest as adrenal insufficiency.

Mars Conjunct Uranus

You are individualistic and crave excitement. You may have difficulty handling stress, so you are prone to stress-related ailments such as headaches or hypertension. You may experience spasms and cramps. You operate at a high energy level, and your high-strung state puts a strain on your nervous system. You are prone to muscle spasms from overtaxing your body. You are adept around machinery and enjoy speed, but there can be accidents around machinery or electrical equipment due to carelessness.

Mars Sextile/Trine Uranus

You have much drive and energy but are prone to nervous tension. You like to try unusual health regimens and can heal quickly from disease. You benefit from high-tech treatments. Your circulation is good, and this aspect aids heart action.

Mars Square/Opposition Uranus

You have an erratic nature, are easily bored, and may crave excitement. You function at high-energy levels and can have difficulty slowing down. At some point in your life you may require surgery. There is a danger of rupture of muscles or spinal problems or lacerations due to pushing yourself too hard. You are easily irritated or frustrated and can find an outlet in sports. Your impulsiveness and liking for danger can lead to accidents or wounds. You are prone to spastic conditions such as pains and cramps from sudden muscle spasms, muscle tics, and fractures. Peppermint tea is helpful for muscle spasms. You should increase your intake of vitamins and minerals when under stress. Use care around appliances, as you are prone to accidents from electrical equipment or damaged insulation. You should avoid highly spiced foods, as your stomach may contain excess hydrochloric acid, creating the potential for an ulcer.

Mars Conjunct Neptune

You are sensitive and idealistic, with a strong desire to help others. This can sometimes be to the detriment of your own health, as you let others rob you of your energy. You need to consume a healthy diet, as you are prone to vitality problems, and you need quiet moments of rest and relaxation. You need to build up your immune system by having a diet containing plenty of fresh fruits and vegetables. You may be allergic to toxins in the air.

Mars Sextile/Trine Neptune

You instinctively follow a proper diet regimen but need to exercise more, as you have a tendency toward flabbiness. You need to drink sufficient water every day to flush out toxins and may benefit from water therapies such as swimming or bathing. A day at the ocean can be revitalizing. There is the potential for faith healing.

Mars Square/Opposition Neptune

You may have poor vitality and a lack of energy. You are prone to stress-related ailments and tend to be drug-sensitive, with a propensity for allergies. The adrenal glands can be weak, leading to adrenal insufficiency. Lack of exercise leads to flabbiness and lack of body tone. You are subject to misdiagnosis and should always get a second opinion on any medical diagnosis. There is also the danger of receiving the wrong medication or treatment or taking an overdose of medicine.

You are susceptible to infections and need to build up your immune system. You are susceptible to pneumonia. You benefit from herbs such as red clover and foods such as wheatgrass, raw carrots and beets, black currants, carrot juice, and citrus fruits. These promote healthy blood. Your muscles tend to be weak and flaccid and would benefit from a regular program of exercise using weights of some type. You are susceptible to adverse reactions from taking large doses of minerals, especially selenium, and can also be susceptible to air pollution. Vitamin E is an aid against a polluted environment. You could be allergic to chlorine.

Mars Conjunct Pluto

You are endowed with tremendous energy, and it is difficult for others to keep up with you. There is a tendency to push yourself to the limits, leading to burnout or muscle injury. Constantly pushing your body to its limits can cause a breakdown of health as you age unless you allow yourself sufficient rest and relaxation. You need some form of exercise to release tension. Dancing and gymnastics might be enjoyable. There is generally resistance to disease and the ability to regenerate yourself.

Mars Sextile/Trine Pluto

You have vitality and endurance and the energy to overcome and transform health problems. You have more energy than average, which helps you take on difficult tasks. In fact, you thrive on hard work. You have healthy reproductive and eliminative systems.

Mars Square/Opposition Pluto

You are subject to stress-related ailments, nervous irritation, and damage to muscles and tendons from pushing yourself too hard. There can be disorders related to the endocrine gland. Mars-Pluto combinations can indicate massive infection, so you may experience inflammatory or feverish responses during illness. Juices made from carrots, beets, lemons, oranges, green pepper, watercress, and parsley strengthen the immune system. There can be blood-related ailments such as blood poisoning or anemia and also the potential for bowel disorders. Foods high in iron, such as apples, beets, apricots, broccoli, blueberries, raisins, spinach, whole wheat, almonds, dates, and wheat germ, are beneficial to prevent anemia, and they contain fiber to aid the bowels. You are prone to parasitic-type ailments such as Lyme disease and should wear protective clothing when in the woods. There can be danger from bee stings. You should increase your intake of minerals when under stress. At some point in your life you might require surgery. In extreme cases, this aspect can indicate an organ transplant. Men with this aspect are prone to inflammation of the prostate. Foods high in zinc, such as pumpkin seeds and sunflower seeds, aid the prostate.

Jupiter Aspects

Jupiter Conjunct Saturn

This aspect occurs every twenty years and can emphasize disorders affecting the sign the planets tenant. (See chapter 2 for more information on the signs in medical astrology.) In general, this aspect can indicate liver dysfunction or gallbladder problems. You may have problems with fat assimilation. Cholesterol levels can be high and should be checked by your doctor.

Jupiter Sextile/Trine Saturn

This aspect confers the discipline necessary for good health. You are able to adopt a healthy regimen of diet and exercise and are willing to forgo excesses in the diet, which are a detriment to good health. The digestive processes function well. This aspect promotes a healthy gallbladder and liver function.

Jupiter Square/Opposition Saturn

There can be nutritional deficiencies due to poor assimilation of vitamins and minerals in the body. You need to ingest healthy oils and forgo fried foods, which can have a deleterious effect on your body. This is due in some cases to exposure to rancid oil and your difficulty in fat assimilation. This aspect can indicate weakened liver function, hardening of the arteries, and problems with the gallbladder. Carrot, beet, and cucumber juices cleanse the gallbladder. Supplements such as acidophilus, activated charcoal, and calcium can help lower cholesterol levels. The hips are a sensitive area, and there is proneness to sciatica. Garlic and iodine are helpful against sciatica. There is the potential for a hernia.

Jupiter Conjunct Uranus

You are an independent person with a sense of adventure. You enjoy trying new techniques and, when ill, can benefit from unusual healing techniques. You have a lot of nervous tension, which can be released through exercise. You have some tendency toward erratic functioning of the liver.

Jupiter Sextile/Trine Uranus

You are spontaneous and creative. You like to keep up with the latest health trends. You like to experiment and will try a new procedure if you think it will aid your health. When ill, there can be the potential for spontaneous healing.

Jupiter Square/Opposition Uranus

You are subject to stress-related conditions, which can find a release through such activities as meditation, yoga, or exercise. There can be spasm conditions in the body, cramping, and a potential for sugar-related problems. You might benefit from extra chromium in your diet. Your metabolism tends to be erratic, and there can be acute liver dysfunction. Your high-strung nature can lead to intestinal disorders.

Jupiter Conjunct Neptune

You are sensitive and idealistic, with a spiritual attitude toward life. Your oversensitive nature makes you prone to allergens in the air. There can be a water imbalance in the body, leading to excess fluid in the tissues. You need to get more exercise, as the muscles can become weakened from lack of use, and there is a tendency toward flabbiness or waterlogged tissues. There can be weakened liver function and a difficulty in fat assimilation.

Jupiter Sextile/Trine Neptune

You are idealistic and sensitive, with a desire to help others. Your natural spiritual attunement to the universe is an aid to good health. You enjoy water therapies such as swimming or bathing. You do best on a diet of natural foods.

Jupiter Square/Opposition Neptune

You may have muscle weakness and a tendency toward flabbiness due to a lack of body tone. You benefit from building up your muscles through the use of weights. You are prone to infections, blood disorders, and liver dysfunction. You have escapist tendencies, which can lead to excessive intake of alcohol or drugs. There can be intestinal disorders. The metabolism is weak, so food is not properly digested, which could lead to abdominal distention. Drinking a combination of lemon juice and water each morning helps improve digestion. You are prone to disorders that may have a psychological origin. There can be misdiagnosis of illness. There is the danger of accidents from gas or fumes, drugs, or chemicals.

Jupiter Conjunct Pluto

You are a person of powerful ambition, with strong regenerative abilities. You have a tendency to do things on a grand scale, and you also tend to have a large appetite. This can lead to diseases caused by excess. There can be a difficulty in fat assimilation.

Jupiter Sextile/Trine Pluto

You have tremendous vitality and regenerative ability. Your nutrition is good, and you have healthy blood. This aspect favors such things as a successful blood transfusion and organ regeneration.

Jupiter Square/Opposition Pluto

You are a person of tremendous appetite to the point of gluttony. There can be compulsive eating, leading to weight gain and liver toxicity. You are also subject to infectious diseases. Your metabolism can be erratic, and you are subject to metabolic disorders. You are prone to infections and should be sure to get proper inoculations before traveling to exotic places.

Saturn Aspects

Saturn Conjunct Uranus

You are prone to psychological tension due to a conflict between your desire for security and your desire for excitement. This can lead to stress-related ailments that involve cramps or spasms. There is the potential for a fracture of a bone or problems with the electrical system of the heart.

Saturn Sextile/Trine Uranus

You are able to combine the best of the old with the new and to deal with stress in a healthy manner. When tense, you find ways to relax such as meditation or yoga. You are scientifically oriented and like to keep up with the latest in medical discoveries. The body has good oxygenation processes.

Saturn Square/Opposition Uranus

You can be tense and irritable. You have difficulty handling stress, which can manifest as contractions and seizures or sudden skin eruptions. There is the potential for injury to the bones or joints. There can be dental disorders. You are subject to chronic diseases such as arthritis. There can be circulatory disorders and nervous complaints.

Saturn Conjunct Neptune

You have a tendency to worry and can fret about nonessentials. You may experience anxiety and low self-esteem, leading to depression. There can be emotional inhibition and neurosis. The organs associated with the signs occupied by both Saturn and Neptune are weak and need to be nourished. (See chapter 4 for an explanation of the planets in the signs.) This aspect refers to chronic disease and gives the potential for chronic illness. The lungs and liver are vulnerable and need to be built up. Smoking cigarettes should be avoided. Liver ailments could be helped by supplementing your diet with lecithin and aloe vera and eating foods such as apples, carrots, zucchini, goat's milk, and raw and unsalted nuts and seeds. There can be a difficulty in fat assimilation and problems with the skin or bowels due to a lack of oils. The bones can be weak, and you benefit from foods high in calcium.

Saturn Sextile/Trine Neptune

You are practical and idealistic. You enjoy eating natural foods and are able to maintain a balanced diet. You have patience and a spiritual outlook, which aids your emotional well-being. When ill, you may benefit from therapies that utilize music or color.

Saturn Square/Opposition Neptune

You are prone to long-term ailments or genetic or hereditary weaknesses. There is lowered immunity and the potential for infectious diseases. You have a tendency toward worry and anxiety, which can lead to neuroses or phobias. You become depressed easily. You are prone to environmental sensitivities such as heavy metal poisoning and can experience respiratory and food allergies and toxicity from prescription drugs. Your system is sensitive to fluoridation and chlorine. Ginger is an excellent detoxifier. Your bones can be weak, giving you a proneness to diseases such as osteoporosis and osteomalacia. You benefit from having a bone scan once you reach middle age.

You have a problem assimilating fats, which may be related to liver dysfunction. High-quality proteins such as goat's milk, brewer's yeast, cottage cheese, and nut butters aid liver function. You are prone to lung diseases such as pneumonia or emphysema, as well as rheumatic diseases. The lungs are helped by flaxseed tea, comfrey,[1] wintergreen tea, and sufficient vitamin C. Thyme is also helpful for lung problems. There can be a psychic component to disease. You need adequate rest, a healthy diet, exercise, and a positive attitude to maintain your health.

Saturn Conjunct Pluto

You may have had weak vitality or undeveloped organs as a child and contracted childhood illnesses. This has helped you become stronger, with more endurance as you age. You can work hard and withstand stress. In fact, you thrive on hard work, which in your case aids your health. You are susceptible to metal poisoning, which can be relieved by vitamin C.

Saturn Sextile/Trine Pluto

You have tenacity and endurance. Your have a solid bone structure and the vitality to withstand periods of stress. You thrive on hard work and are highly disciplined. You enjoy strenuous exercise and tend toward a modest diet.

Saturn Square/Opposition Pluto

You have a sensitive body and are prone to chronic diseases. There can be a tendency toward hardening or calcification in the body. Your digestion can be poor, with a tendency toward bowel disorders, causing you to retain metabolic wastes. This increases body toxicity. Ginger is an excellent detoxifier. You are subject to metal poisoning and should increase your intake of vitamin C. The bones are vulnerable, and there is a potential for bone injuries. Physical exercise helps build up the bones. You can also benefit from dairy products such as yogurt, kefir, and buttermilk as well as foods high in minerals such as sea vegetables, whole grains, and cabbage. You are highly sensitive to pollution and do better in a clean atmosphere. There can be blood disorders such as anemia. Foods high in iron, such as apples, beets, apricots, broccoli, blueberries, raisins, spinach, whole wheat, almonds, dates, and wheat germ, are beneficial to prevent anemia.

Uranus Aspects

The planets Uranus, Neptune, and Pluto move so slowly that many people are born with the following aspects. These are considered generational aspects. One would need more confirmation from other planetary combinations before making a judgment based on these planets in combination with each other.

Uranus Conjunct Neptune

You can be high-strung and nervous. You have a tendency to overreact, putting a strain on your nervous system. There can be an imbalance in the rhythmic processes of your body, which are aided by maintaining a daily routine of diet and exercise. There is some potential for breathing disorders and allergies.

Uranus Sextile/Trine Neptune

You have a positive attitude and a balanced approach to diet and exercise. You tend toward moderation in your diet and rarely abuse drugs or alcohol. You are interested in learning about new health routines.

Uranus Square/Opposition Neptune

You can be nervous and high-strung and have problems handling stress. There can be a desire to escape the harsh realities of life, causing a dependency on drugs or alcohol. Your bodily rhythms can be off, as you do not wish to follow any kind of diet or exercise routine. There can be breathing problems or circulatory disorders.

Uranus Conjunct Pluto

You can be nervous and high-strung and are prone to stress-related ailments. This can be in the form of spastic conditions or heart palpitations. There is a need for moderation in the diet, as there can be body toxicity from improper nutrition. Ginger is an excellent detoxifier.

Uranus Sextile/Trine Pluto

You are innovative and adventurous. Your body is healthy, and you are able to eliminate toxins from your body and regenerate yourself. You have good oxygenation processes in your body.

Uranus Square/Opposition Pluto

You are prone to exaggeration and immoderation. You are easily excitable and do not handle stress well. It is difficult for you to follow a healthy diet regimen. You are prone to nervous or breathing disorders. Nervousness can lead to tics or spastic conditions.

Neptune Aspects

Neptune-Pluto aspects occur for long periods of time and affect whole generations. They are unlikely to have any effect on an individual's health.

---

1. Comfrey is best used externally as an ointment or as tincture drops in water made into a compress. Do not ingest, as some studies suggest that comfrey is carcinogenic in large doses.

6
The Houses in Medical Astrology

As you can see from your birth chart, there are twelve houses in a horoscope. The houses operate on many levels but generally describe where the actions indicated by a particular planet take place. A house is colored by planets that occupy or rule it and by the sign on its cusp. Sometimes one or more houses in a chart are emphasized by being occupied by two or more planets. This can be an area of life that has great significance to you. For example, using natal astrology, if you have two or more planets in the tenth house of profession, there can be an interest in or an emphasis on career goals. Your reputation is important to you, and, depending on which planets occupy the house, you may receive recognition or become an authority in a particular area.

In medical astrology, an emphasis of planets in a house would pertain more to the parts of the body that it relates to in the natural zodiac. For example, since the first sign of the zodiac is Aries, the first house always has a connection with Aries-ruled parts of the body—the head, face, upper jaw, etc. (See chapter 2 for more information on the signs in medical astrology.)

The physiology or function of a planet in a house describes its action in connection with the parts of body that the house represents. For example, if Mars is found in your fourth house, you might be prone to stomach upset or an acid stomach. The fourth house is the natural house of the sign Cancer, which is associated with the stomach. Since Mars rules inflammation, there is the potential for an inflammatory stomach disorder. Knowing this, you can take preventive action to avoid stressing the stomach.

As another example, Pluto in the eighth house could indicate potential bowel disorders. Pluto is the natural ruler of the eighth house, which refers to the sign Scorpio, which is associated with the eliminative organs. These would be vulnerable parts of the body that need to be kept in good working order and need your attention.

The interpretations that follow are limited to a planet in a house and do not take into account other factors in the chart. They are informative but are not the final word on any health disorder or weakness indicated by the chart. The houses should be used as part of a complete health interpretation in judging bodily weakness and proneness to specific disease states. For example, if one has determined that there is a weakness in the kidney area, then an emphasis of planets in the seventh house, the natural house of Libra, which is associated with the kidneys, could be a further indication. An emphasis in the fifth and eleventh houses could be an indication of circulatory disorders. As you will see, the fifth and eleventh houses are associated with the heart and circulation. An emphasis in the third and ninth houses could be a factor in respiratory disorders, as the third and ninth houses are associated with respiratory disorders.

The houses can reveal an environmental factor that affects health. There can be functional disorders relating to the natural ruler of that house. The houses are divided into angular, succedent, and cadent houses. The angular houses are houses one, four, seven, and ten; the succedent houses are houses two, five, eight, and eleven; and the cadent houses are houses three, six, nine, and twelve.

In general, an emphasis of planets in angular houses can describe someone who likes to live an active life and who can be direct and outgoing. The parts of the body affected relate to the cardinal mode and are described more fully in chapter 9. There is a tendency to push oneself too hard, leading to a potential breakdown in health. The parts of the body affected by the succedent houses relate to the fixed mode and are also described in chapter 9. An emphasis in these houses can indicate a rigid and obsessive personality, leading to stiff muscles and joints and potential mobility problems. An emphasis in the cadent houses relates to the mutable mode and are also described in chapter 9. This can describe a person who experiences nervous or respiratory disorders and who can be high-strung and anxious.

House Descriptions in Medical Astrology

The following descriptions of each house are followed by examples of the planets in each of the houses.

First House

The first house is descriptive of the personality and the physical body. It can describe one's appearance and physical vitality. It can also describe one's early development and environmental issues that affect the personality and physical body. (See the first part of chapter 7 for an interpretation of your Ascendant, which is the sign on your first-house cusp.)

A first-house emphasis (two or more planets in a house) can give a strong personality and leadership ability. There is an urgent need to express oneself. It is the natural house of Aries, and individuals with this emphasis tend to have a competitive nature and be aggressive, with a desire to be first. This can strain one physically and mentally. First-house individuals rarely slow down. There is a need to learn how to conserve energy, as it is rapidly depleted by misuse. If one does not learn to practice moderation, the body can eventually break down from driving it too hard.

The first house rules the head, so it is associated with head injuries, fevers, and headaches. It is also connected with dizzy spells, dental disorders, and hearing problems. It is sometimes associated with mental disorders and stroke.

Second House

The second house is the natural house of Taurus, a sign having to do with the senses. It is therefore descriptive of one's food tastes.

Briefly, Aries on the second-house cusp indicates someone who likes hot and spicy foods; Taurus likes rich food and may overeat sweets; Gemini likes variety in food; Cancer likes the so-called comfort foods; Leo has a liking for rich and heavy foods and high-quality food; Virgo may have a tendency to eat natural foods and can be a fussy eater; Libra likes rich food and also may crave sweets; Scorpio likes a meal high in proteins and can overdo red meat; Sagittarius has a liking for rich food, especially food high in fat; Capricorn likes high-quality foods and proteins; Aquarius likes to try unusual foods and can be eccentric in food tastes; and Pisces enjoys seafood, soups, and stews. Needless to say, one's taste preferences can be modified by one's Sun sign and other planetary placements.

An emphasis of planets in the second house could indicate a craving for sugar and a difficulty in metabolizing sugar, leading to diseases such as hypoglycemia or diabetes. There could also be a rigidity and stubbornness to the personality. Disorders involving sense deprivation would be found here. The second house is also associated with disorders affecting the neck and throat.

Third House

The third house is the natural house of Gemini, a sign of communication, the mind, and mobility. An emphasis of planets in this house could indicate potential respiratory disorders, a hormonal imbalance, and mobility problems. There can be mental disorders or nervousness and anxiety. There could also be environmental allergies. An overactive mind can lead to insomnia.

Fourth House

The fourth house is the natural house of Cancer. This house is associated with eating disorders such as bulimia or anorexia. There can be digestive disorders, and in females there can be problems related to the breast or womb. The fourth house is associated with nutrition. Therefore, problems with overeating or a lack of appetite would be found here. This house is part of the parental axis and may refer to the mother, with the tenth house referring to the father. Psychological problems stemming from early childhood or a lack of nurturing may be seen here.

Fifth House

The fifth house is the natural house of Leo. When any of the so-called stressful planets (Mars, Saturn, Uranus, Neptune, or Pluto) occupy this house or its opposite house, the eleventh house, there can be problems with the heart and circulation, leading to heart disease. This house is also associated with childbirth, and along with other factors in the chart is an indication of the ability or inability to conceive. Back and spinal problems may show up in this house.

Sixth House

The sixth house, which is the natural house of Virgo, is called the house of health. Since this house traditionally refers to health in the natal chart, it is worth examining the sign on the cusp of your sixth-house cusp. See the last part of chapter 7 for an in-depth analysis of the sign found on the cusp of your sixth house.

The sixth house is concerned with the efficient running of your body through diet and exercise and can indicate functional disorders, disturbances of your daily routine leading to illness, and harmful working conditions that affect the body. It can describe sickness due to overwork or poor assimilation of food that causes nutritional deficiencies. Planets in the sixth house can indicate allergies, mental disorders, sugar metabolism problems, or digestive upsets. Sometimes an emphasis of planets in this house can indicate an unhealthy obsession with health or hypochondriacal tendencies.

Seventh House

The seventh house is the natural house of Libra and is thus related to the action of the kidneys. It refers to balance, and a concentration of planets here can indicate a potential imbalance of energy in the body or kidney dysfunction. There can also be problems with the lower back.

Eighth House

The eighth house is the natural house of Scorpio. A heavy concentration of planets in this house adds an intensity to the personality and can result in many tests on the body and potential psychological problems. An emphasis of planets in this house can describe someone who is strong and forceful, with deep emotional scars. There is a need to transform and regenerate the body. This house is also referred to as the house of sex. Unhealthy sexual practices can lead to venereal diseases or sexual obsession.

With a concentration of planets in the eighth house, one can have a tendency to push the body too hard. The emotions run deep, and there are extremes in the personality. You can be helped by psychological counseling. Physically, there can be bowel disorders or diseases associated with the colon such as diverticulitis or colitis.

Ninth House

The ninth house is the natural house of Sagittarius. Being opposite the third house, there can be respiratory disorders and weak lungs. There can be breathing problems. With Sagittarius ruling the hips and thighs, one may be susceptible to disorders such as sciatica and locomotor problems. The ninth house is also associated with travel, and therefore any illness or accident related to travel.

Tenth House

The tenth house is the natural house of Capricorn. An emphasis of planets in this house can describe someone who is susceptible to societal pressures. There can be a desire to be at the top no matter what the cost. This puts the body under great stress, and one may not take enough time to rest and relax. The tenth house is linked to the knees, bones, and joints, as well as to calcium metabolism and the function of the gallbladder. With an emphasis here, there can be excess cholesterol and sluggish bile production.

Eleventh House

The eleventh house is the natural house of Aquarius. This house works in tandem with the fifth house and rules the heart and circulation. An emphasis of planets in this house can indicate circulatory disorders and problems with the lower legs. The eleventh house is associated with future goals, and an emphasis here describes someone who needs to face the future with hope and optimism.

Twelfth House

The twelfth house is the natural house of Pisces. An emphasis of planets here can describe someone who is introverted and may have psychological problems. There can be a subconscious influence on the personality. You can build up negative emotions until there is a physical manifestation of disease. You may benefit from therapy and facing your problems realistically. This house is associated with autoimmune diseases and a need to build up the immune system.

The Planets in the Houses in Medical Astrology

The following is a description of the each of the planets in the twelve houses of the birth chart. The energy of the planet is combined with the nature of the house to describe a potential strength or weakness in the body. The information summarizes basic tendencies. You will gain more information by examining the specific aspects made to each planet. It should always be kept in mind that it takes more than one combination to indicate a specific disorder. When difficulties are indicated by a planet, it is usually because the planet is receiving a difficult or stressful aspect. You can examine all of your planetary aspects and determine the relative strength or weakness of the aspects made to a particular planet by seeing if the planet receives a majority of favorable or unfavorable aspects. See chapter 5 for an interpretation of the aspects in your chart in relation to medical astrology. See Appendix B: How to Use This Book for help in finding your aspects. Information to help prevent or treat the bodily weaknesses mentioned in the following interpretations has been touched on in previous chapters. See also Appendix A: Nutritional Guidance to Nourish Weak Areas of the Body for more information.

The Sun in the Houses

Sun in the First House

You have a strong personality and are considered energetic and courageous. You have the ability to fight disease and recuperate quickly from illness. You benefit from physical exercise, as this will increase your stamina.

Sun in the Second House

You have a strong hold on life and much physical endurance. You have strength in your upper body and can gain more strength through weightlifting. You are able to rejuvenate yourself through contact with nature.

Sun in the Third House

You are mentally alert and enjoy being busy. You easily adjust to new situations and thrive on variety. You may be prone to getting an infection when in contact with masses of people, so avoid large crowds during flu epidemics.

Sun in the Fourth House

You have strength and good resistance to disease. When nervous and upset, you tend toward stomach complaints. Having a secure home and family increases your emotional security and aids your health.

Sun in the Fifth House

You have much vitality and a positive outlook on life. You are fond of children, and this placement favors being a parent. You could have a tendency toward high cholesterol and eventual heart disease if you do not follow a proper diet.

Sun in the Sixth House

You have a strong interest in health and nutrition but a tendency to become obsessed with your body. This can lead to being a hypochondriac. You need to follow a natural diet and exercise regularly, and try to avoid junk food as you have a sensitive constitution. Keeping your bowels in good working order is an aid to good health.

Sun in the Seventh House

You have vitality and resistance to disease. You function best in relationships with others and can become ill from disharmonious relationships. You need to drink plenty of water every day to flush out your kidneys.

Sun in the Eighth House

You are psychologically intense and powerfully driven. You may push your body beyond its limits, leading to a breakdown in the future. You benefit from eating a diet high in fiber to avoid a weakness in the colon area.

Sun in the Ninth House

Your optimistic nature and healthy attitude are aids to good health. Having a religious outlook also aids your health. You like to be on the go, and benefit from outdoor exercise. You have some tendency to overindulge in fats, which puts a strain on your liver.

Sun in the Tenth House

You have strength and vitality and are able to overcome disease. You have a good bone structure, which gives you endurance and mobility. You benefit from eating foods high in calcium.

Sun in the Eleventh House

Your hopeful outlook is an aid to emotional balance. You function best in group situations and remain healthy and emotionally stable when you have goals. At times you can be overly rigid, leading to circulatory problems. You have some tendency to be high-strung.

Sun in the Twelfth House

People may not see you as you really are. As a child you might have been shy and withdrawn. One of your greatest wishes is to serve others. You may have an unconscious desire for power and recognition. The twelfth house has rulership over the immune system, which can be a weak point in your body. You may be subject to colds, flus, and viral infections.

The Moon in the Houses

Moon in the First House

You are emotionally sensitive and can be changeable and moody. You have strong needs and desires, which, if not met, can cause you to withdraw from others. When upset, you can get stomach indigestion or more serious disorders such as acid reflux or stomach ulcers.

Moon in the Second House

You have a strong constitution but some tendency toward laziness. You benefit from a regular exercise regimen as you may have poor muscle tone. Too much of a sweet tooth can cause problems with blood-sugar metabolism.

Moon in the Third House

You have much energy and vitality but tend to run on nervous energy. This can cause you to become high-strung and nervous. You love to be busy and need a lot of mental stimulation. You can have difficulty turning off your mind at night, leading to insomnia. You may be prone to mucus formation in the lungs.

Moon in the Fourth House

Your health depends on your emotional security. If you feel adrift without any roots, you become more susceptible to illness. It is important for you to follow a healthy diet, as you are prone to eating disorders such as anorexia or bulimia. Women with this placement are prone to breast cysts or fibroid tumors.

Moon in the Fifth House

You have a love of and a desire for children. This placement can be an indication of the ability to conceive and have a large family. There can be a love of rich foods, which tend to raise cholesterol levels.

Moon in the Sixth House

You have a strong interest in health, diet, and hygiene. You can become obsessed with your health and develop psychosomatic illnesses. You benefit from a nutritious diet and daily exercise. You need to live a balanced life in order not to disturb your bodily rhythms.

Moon in the Seventh House

Your emotional well-being is dependent on being in a healthy relationship. A disharmonious relationship can make you feel ill. Your tendency toward overindulgence in food and drink can lead to indigestion or diseases caused by excess.

Moon in the Eighth House

You need to keep your reproductive and eliminative organs in good shape in order to ensure good health. You have a tendency toward bowel disorders such as constipation or diarrhea, and the potential for bladder disease. Unhealthy sexual practices can lead to sexually transmitted diseases. You tend toward extremes in emotional behavior.

Moon in the Ninth House

You are a person with vision. Your positive outlook and strong need for mental stimulation are aids to good health. At times, too much mental stimulation can lead to restlessness or a difficulty in turning off the mind at night, leading to bouts of insomnia. There can be some weakness in the hips and thighs, and a craving for fatty foods can put a strain on the liver.

Moon in the Tenth House

You are serious and hard working and have a strong sense of duty. You are sensible and tend to follow a healthy diet. You can be rigid and inflexible, leading to health problems such as arthritis or rheumatism. There can be a propensity toward swollen knees.

Moon in the Eleventh House

You are unique and independent. You have a tendency to overreact emotionally, putting a strain on your nervous system. There can be a weakness in the lower legs, leading to swollen ankles or a sprained ankle.

Moon in the Twelfth House

You have complex emotions and may desire to be alone in order to pursue your creative or spiritual inclinations. You may have a weak constitution and need to build up your immune system. You may have unusual cravings and contract rare or unusual diseases. There can be a water imbalance in the body due to a sodium/potassium imbalance.

Mercury in the Houses

Mercury in the First House

You are a good communicator with a strong desire to express yourself. You are talkative and like to write. You come and go a great deal and may experience nervous exhaustion. There can be a tendency to worry, which can lower resistance, or a difficulty in turning off the mind at night, leading to insomnia.

Mercury in the Second House

You have strong values and can be dogmatic in speech. You are sensitive in the throat and neck area and may experience hoarseness or a sore throat when under stress. You have a good sense of taste and smell.

Mercury in the Third House

You are agile and quick-witted. You enjoy being busy and can handle more than one task at a time. You may run on nervous energy, and need periods of calm to quiet your nerves. You may be prone to respiratory ailments and mental anxiety.

Mercury in the Fourth House

You have a good memory with some tendency to cling to the past. You worry unnecessarily about trivial things, causing potential stomach upsets, indigestion, or pains in the abdomen. You think a lot about food and are a good cook but have a tendency toward overindulgence.

Mercury in the Fifth House

You are creative and have a natural theatrical bent. You desire children and would make a good parent. You enjoy sports and recreation but need to be careful of accidents to your hands or arms.

Mercury in the Sixth House

You are organized and detail-oriented. Chaotic situations can cause you to become ill. You have a strong interest in diet and hygiene and enjoy keeping abreast of the latest health trends. You have a tendency to worry over trifles, which could lead to nervousness and anxiety. You could also be phobic about germs. There can be a weakness in the intestinal area.

Mercury in the Seventh House

You work well in one-to-one situations and are upset easily in disharmonious relationships. This could lead to headaches or skin eruptions. You have a sensitive nervous system, which can manifest as disorders of the sensory nerves.

Mercury in the Eighth House

You are sharp and incisive, with a probing mind that at times borders on obsessiveness. You need to guard against compulsive behavior. There can be damage to the motor nerves in the body and a potential for bowel disorders caused by worry.

Mercury in the Ninth House

You have a broad view of life and need mental stimulation for your emotional well-being. You are prone to respiratory ailments and locomotor disorders. You have a liking for rich food, which can put a strain on the liver.

Mercury in the Tenth House

You are an excellent communicator and enjoy being thought of as an authority. You can become rigid in your views and have stiff joints and disorders such as arthritis or rheumatism. You may experience allergies that manifest as skin disorders.

Mercury in the Eleventh House

You are intelligent and far-sighted. You can be high-strung and run on nervous energy. You are prone to nervous exhaustion, which can lead to tics or twitches. There can be circulatory problems and accidents resulting in a sprained or broken ankle.

Mercury in the Twelfth House

You have a psychic sensitivity and a strong spiritual or creative bent. You benefit from disciplines such as meditation or yoga. Your strong sensitivity can lower your resistance, making you vulnerable to colds and flus. You are susceptible to suggestion as well as to being misdiagnosed, so you should always get a second opinion on any medical diagnosis. You need to practice positive thinking.

Venus in the Houses

Venus in the First House

You have good health and a healthy outlook on life. There is emotional balance and harmony. You have some tendency toward self-indulgence, which can lead to the ill effects from eating foods high in sugar that rob the body of nutrients. You are prone to skin problems such as hives when upset and acne from a poor diet.

Venus in the Second House

You have a strong sensual nature and a good sense of taste and smell. You have a tendency toward self-indulgence in food and drink. You are prone to disorders in the neck and throat area and have a tendency to choke or gag on food.

Venus in the Third House

You are social and gregarious with a natural, creative bent. Your nervous system is sensitive, and there can be a tendency toward respiratory disorders. Excessive talking can lead to hoarseness.

Venus in the Fourth House

You are a gourmet cook who loves to entertain. You overindulge in food and drink, leading to stomach upset as well as guilt at overeating. You may also experience gas or bloating. When upset, you can become nauseous.

Venus in the Fifth House

You are creative and sociable and have an optimistic outlook on life. Your positive attitude is an aid to good health. You are prone to heart palpitations and backaches. There can be circulatory disorders. Women with this placement are usually able to conceive easily.

Venus in the Sixth House

You are kind and generous and tend to have good health. A tendency to overindulge can put a strain on the intestines and lead to bouts of constipation or diarrhea. Your health will be stable if you do not abuse your body through poor diet and lack of exercise.

Venus in the Seventh House

You relate well to others and enjoy socializing. Your well-being is dependent on your being in a harmonious relationship. When upset, you are subject to skin disorders such as a rash or hives. You need to drink plenty of water to continually flush your kidneys.

Venus in the Eighth House

You can be intense and serious in matters of love and sex. Women with this placement are prone to menstrual irregularities and conditions such as cystitis. Sexually transmitted diseases are a potential for both sexes, and can be prevented by practicing safe sex. This placement is considered positive for fertility.

Venus in the Ninth House

You have vitality and high spirits. You enjoy broadening your horizons. You also love to eat and indulge yourself in foods that are high in protein and fat. This can strain both the liver and the kidneys and cause an increase of uric acid in the body, a symptom of gout. There is a propensity toward respiratory ailments or conditions such as sciatica.

Venus in the Tenth House

You have vitality and endurance and are seen by others in a favorable way. There can be a tendency toward skin ailments and stomach disorders when under pressure. You may also be prone to gout from eating a diet too high in protein.

Venus in the Eleventh House

You are friendly and warm and enjoy the company of many friends. Your good nature is a boost to others. You are prone to circulatory ailments and disorders of the blood involving the veins. You need to avoid laziness and sedentary behavior, which increase the risk of circulatory disorders. You tend to overact emotionally and are prone to hysteria. You benefit from exercises to strengthen your lower legs, which are vulnerable areas.

Venus in the Twelfth House

You are creative and spiritual and are able to recharge yourself through times of quiet contemplation or artistic activity. A tendency toward laziness and self-indulgence leads to poor health habits that can depress your vulnerable immune system. There can also be a weakness in the feet.

Mars in the Houses

Mars in the First House

You are active and aggressive. You have a strong constitution and are able to surmount most threats to health. You may take your good health for granted and not take good care of yourself, which could lead to a health breakdown in the future. This is because you have a tendency to drive yourself too hard, causing burnout. You may not get sufficient rest, and you need to slow down and learn moderation. Your impetuousness can lead to accidents, especially to the head. Your aggressive nature can find a healthy outlet in physical exercise and outdoor sports.

Mars in the Second House

You have good endurance and a strong constitution. There can be a propensity toward dental troubles, especially in the gum area. There can also be polyps in the nose that can obstruct breathing. Be sure to chew your food completely, as you are susceptible to choking on your food. You may also get frequent sore throats and pain in the neck area.

Mars in the Third House

You are a good communicator and enjoy being busy. You may have a high-strung temperament, leading to nervous disorders. You tend to be a fast driver. This could lead to accidents causing whiplash. You need to be careful when using sharp instruments or in sports activities, as there can be a tendency toward cuts, bruises, or sprains involving the arms, hands, and wrists. There is danger of slipping on ice in cold weather. You also have a tendency to overstrain your muscles by lifting heavy objects. You are prone to repetitive-motion disorders such as carpal tunnel syndrome.

Mars in the Fourth House

You are emotionally active and have a good constitution. You can get upset easily, leading to stomach upset and indigestion. You have a tendency to worry too much, which undermines your health and can lead to conditions such as stomach ulcers. There can be a tendency to feverish and inflammatory disorders. You are prone to accidents in the home, so you should use care around sharp objects and appliances. You should also be careful around stoves, as there is the danger of burns and scalds.

Mars in the Fifth House

You have much vitality and endurance. You benefit from physical exercise but have a tendency to overexert and strain yourself, leading to a potential back injury. You should watch your diet, especially fat intake, as you have a tendency toward heart trouble. It would be wise to have your cholesterol levels checked on a regular basis.

Mars in the Sixth House

You are a hard worker and can be mechanically inclined. Constant overwork leads to tension and irritability. You can injure yourself from overdoing it at work, or there can be accidents while at work. When ill, you are prone to inflammatory diseases or infections. There is the potential for surgery at some point in your life and high fevers when ill.

Mars in the Seventh House

You can be aggressive and outgoing. You have stamina and endurance. When ill, there can be high fevers and a potential for kidney inflammation. Upsets in relationships can lead to stomach disorders, headaches, and skin eruptions. You should cover your head when in direct sunlight, as you are susceptible to sunstroke.

Mars in the Eighth House

You are intense and can be willful and dogmatic. You have a tendency to push yourself too hard, which can lead to a breakdown in health. There is a need to learn moderation. You are prone to bowel and urinary disorders and can have problems with your reproductive system. You can experience wounds or cuts from accidental conditions. You have a strong sex drive and need to use proper precautions to avoid sexually transmitted diseases.

Mars in the Ninth House

You are optimistic and outgoing and like to be on the go. You have good vitality and resistance to disease. It is important that you use caution while traveling, as there is the potential for falling or accidents to the hips and thighs. You are also prone to injuries around horses. There can also be inflammatory disorders involving the hips and thighs, such as sciatica.

Mars in the Tenth House

You are ambitious and active, and have a reserve of energy that keeps you on the go. There is vitality and resistance to disease. When under stress or upset, you may get ailments such as skin eruptions or stomach disorders. You are also prone to more serious skin conditions such as psoriasis or eczema. An improper diet can lead to disorders such as gout, which would probably manifest as an arthritic condition in your knees.

Mars in the Eleventh House

You are outgoing and desire the unusual and unique. You can be high-strung and temperamental and overstrain your nervous system. Pushing yourself too hard and not allowing time for rest and relaxation can lead to a nervous breakdown. You can be prone to circulatory disorders and heart palpitations. You should use care when walking on wet or icy sidewalks, as there is the danger of accidents causing injuries to your lower legs and ankles.

Mars in the Twelfth House

You enjoy creative and spiritual activities, which aid your emotional well-being. You have a sensitive immune system, with a propensity toward infectious disorders and contracting flus and colds. The lungs are sensitive, and you should keep the chest area warm. There can be accidents causing injury to the feet, or foot disorders such as corns or bunions. There can be blood disorders such as anemia.

Jupiter in the Houses

Jupiter in the First House

You are optimistic and generous, and have good health and vitality. You tend toward extravagance and exaggeration. There can be overindulgence in food and drink, and diseases caused by excess. Health problems are caused by toxins in the blood. A love of eating can cause weight gain, especially in the later years. The liver can be a sensitive part of the body.

Jupiter in the Second House

You have a healthy body with much endurance. You have a hearty appetite, which can lead to overindulgence in rich foods. There can be swollen glands in the neck area. You may have difficulty metabolizing sugar, creating a tendency toward hypoglycemia or diabetes. You have a tendency to accumulate fat in the neck area.

Jupiter in the Third House

You are energetic and robust, self-expressive and active. The lungs are a sensitive area, and there can also be a tendency toward tonsillitis. There can be swellings in the hips or thighs. The liver is also a sensitive part of your body.

Jupiter in the Fourth House

You have an expansive and generous nature. You have vitality and longevity. You are prone to stomach upset when overindulging and may also have flatulence from improper eating habits. You have some tendency to gorge yourself on food, which can lead to stomach cramping and nausea.

Jupiter in the Fifth House

You have vitality and optimism but a tendency toward self-indulgence. You gain strength through exercise and self-control. The heart can be a sensitive area, and you are disposed toward high cholesterol. You need to watch your fat intake. There can be diseases caused by excess, leading to toxin-filled blood.

Jupiter in the Sixth House

You have good health and a sturdy body, but you also have a tendency to overindulge in food and drink, leading to weight gain. The liver is a sensitive area. You should try to avoid foods containing hydrogenated oils. The lungs as well as the intestinal area can be sensitive. You need plenty of raw foods to promote enzyme action in your body.

Jupiter in the Seventh House

You tend toward good health and longevity. The kidneys can be a sensitive area, and there can be headaches or skin eruptions from poor kidney function. There can also be episodes of dizziness or vertigo. Insufficient adrenal activity can lead to depression.

Jupiter in the Eighth House

You have good health and longevity. You are sensible in your diet and practice moderation. There is the ability to regenerate your body and improve after illness. The reproductive and eliminative organs are sensitive areas, and men with this placement are prone to an enlarged prostate. Both sexes are prone to sexual excess, which needs to be curbed to avoid sexually transmitted diseases.

Jupiter in the Ninth House

You have an optimistic and hopeful attitude, which is an aid to good health. Your health improves with outdoor exercise, especially walking, as there is a tendency for fat to accumulate on your hips and thighs. You also tend to overindulge in food and drink, which can lead to diseases caused by excess. The hip and thigh area is sensitive and prone to injury.

Jupiter in the Tenth House

You have good vitality and endurance. You can gain greater strength by engaging in activities such as swimming and outdoor activities and getting sufficient sunlight. There can be a tendency toward digestive ailments and skin eruptions. Eating too many fatty foods can put a strain on the liver. Cholesterol levels should be checked regularly.

Jupiter in the Eleventh House

Your hopeful outlook and faith in the future are aids to both emotional and physical health. You enjoy the company of close friends, who in turn feel good in your presence. The circulatory system is sensitive, and there is a need to avoid eating fatty foods that clog the arteries. You may also experience swollen ankles.

Jupiter in the Twelfth House

Your strong faith and spiritual attitude give you courage and hope. You are able to overcome illness and can find yourself spiritually healed. The immune system is sensitive and needs to be built up. You can experience swollen lymph glands and need to be on a diet that cleanses the lymph glands. The spleen is also a sensitive area.

Saturn in the Houses

Saturn in the First House

You have strength and endurance and a mature sense of responsibility but may have contracted early childhood illnesses. There may have been some deprivation or neglect in your formative years, leading to skin disorders, thinning hair, and dental problems. You may also get headaches and have insufficient adrenal activity. A somber attitude can lead to depression.

Saturn in the Second House

You have a strong sense of self-worth and are willing to work hard to make your way in life. When tense, you may develop a stiff neck, which can be helped by massage. There can be a weakness in the gum area and the potential for periodontal disease. The thyroid can be underactive, leading to weight gain or depression. You are prone to sore throats and weak tonsils. There can be constriction of the throat when tired or upset.

Saturn in the Third House

You are a deep thinker who is structured and organized. You can be anxious about your abilities and become depressed easily. Insecurities about your communicative ability may lead to stammering or stuttering. The lungs and respiratory system are particularly vulnerable, and you should avoid smoking or being around secondhand smoke. You are subject to falls. There can also be a proneness to a hearing debility.

Saturn in the Fourth House

You are security-conscious and seek the safety of a home and family. There could have been a loss in your early childhood, causing a basic insecurity. You can be psychologically vulnerable and develop an eating disorder that has its roots in early childhood. The stomach is a weak area, and you are vulnerable to stomach upset caused by anxiety. Women with this placement may have a weakness in the breast and womb areas.

Saturn in the Fifth House

You are serious-minded and are not one to waste time on frivolous activities. The heart and circulatory areas are sensitive, and it is important that you watch your diet, as you may have a tendency toward high cholesterol. You may enjoy outdoor sports but need to be careful as you could strain your back. Women with this placement may experience prolonged labor during childbirth or a difficult pregnancy.

Saturn in the Sixth House

You need to pay attention to your health throughout your lifetime, as sickness can be due to neglect. You are prone to health problems due to worry or overwork. Living as structured a lifestyle as possible is an aid to good health. You do better in a warm climate and should avoid dampness or cold environments, which can lower your vitality and lead to colds and flus. You can be susceptible to aching joints and illnesses such as arthritis and rheumatism. It is important that you avoid toxins in the workplace, as you are subject to industrial diseases. The stomach is also a weak area, and there is a proneness to ailments such as appendicitis. You are subject to falls.

Saturn in the Seventh House

You can be serious and austere. You are able to discipline yourself in matters of health and enjoy a well-regulated life. You are subject to lower back pain when under stress. There can be a weakness in the kidney area and the potential for kidney stones. You need to drink plenty of water to keep the kidneys flushed. You may also be subject to skin diseases and may lack sufficient oil in your diet.

Saturn in the Eighth House

You have endurance and discipline. You need to eat a healthy diet with plenty of fruits, vegetables, and whole grains to keep the eliminative organs functioning. You may have a tendency toward constipation, hemorrhoids, or other bowel disorders. There is also a tendency toward nasal catarrh. There can be an underfunctioning of the sexual organs. Women with this placement may have menstrual disorders. Men can have a weakness in the prostate area.

Saturn in the Ninth House

You have a strong philosophy of life, which guides your actions. You are a lover of tradition and believe in old-fashioned health remedies when ill. You have some tendency toward locomotor disorders and are prone to accidents involving the hands, arms, and legs. There can be some tendency toward high cholesterol levels, which should be checked on a regular basis.

Saturn in the Tenth House

You are authoritative and disciplined, with much endurance. You are able to follow a strict diet and a healthy exercise regimen, which promotes good health. There is a weakness in the bones and teeth, and you need to schedule regular visits to a dentist, as you are prone to tooth decay. A bone density test when older can give you a clue as to whether there is any bone weakness in your body. You may be subject to aching joints and arthritis in the knees. When it comes to treating a health disorder, you prefer the tried and true and will avoid nontraditional forms of healing.

Saturn in the Eleventh House

You are serious-minded and disciplined. You are able to apply the latest scientific discoveries to improving your health. There can be a weakness in the heart and circulatory areas. You are subject to valvular heart trouble. There can be a weakness in the lower legs and ankles and a susceptibility to a sprained or broken ankle. You may also experience tension-related ailments.

Saturn in the Twelfth House

You work well when alone and at times seem to thrive on isolation. Your immune system can be weak and needs to be built up. There can be a weakness in the foot area and conditions such as foot deformity, fallen arches, bunions, cold feet, and accidents causing injury to the feet. You have a tendency toward worry and anxiety, which can lead to depression. There is a need to cultivate a positive attitude.

Uranus in the Houses

Uranus in the First House

You have an exciting, scintillating personality. You are highly independent and are always ready for the new. However, you can be restless, high-strung, and willful. You can be accident-prone, causing injuries to the head from machinery. You can experience spasmodic disorders and cramps. There is the potential for rupture of a tissue. The rhythmic process of your body can be uneven, and it can be difficult for you to live a regulated life. Sudden changes in your life bring stress-related ailments such as headaches and stomach cramps or hypertension. There can also be sudden surgery.

Uranus in the Second House

You have unusual eating tastes and an erratic diet. There can be sudden changes in blood sugar levels in your body, leading to a potential for diabetes or hypoglycemia. When under stress, you can lose your voice suddenly. There can be a disturbance in the venous circulation of your body, leading to conditions such as varicose veins or phlebitis.

Uranus in the Third House

You have a unique mind and are scientifically oriented. You tend to be mentally overactive, leading to bouts of insomnia and nervousness. Your nervous system is highly sensitive, and you need sufficient rest. There can be sudden breathing problems or attacks of asthma. You should take precautions when using heavy machinery and should avoid speeding while driving, as impetuous behavior can lead to accidents.

Uranus in the Fourth House

You enjoy an unusual home life and tend toward an erratic diet. Unhealthy eating can lead to eating disorders and malnutrition. When under stress, you can experience stomach cramps or ulcers. Highly spiced food can upset your stomach, which is slightly acidic. There is the danger of accidents in the home, especially around electricity or involving electrical appliances.

Uranus in the Fifth House

You are creative and enjoy unusual activities. There can be a weakness in the heart and circulatory areas, leading to such disorders as poor circulation, heart palpitations, or cardiovascular disease. Women with this placement are subject to miscarriage or unexpected pregnancy. Be careful of lifting heavy objects, as you have a tendency for sudden and severe back pain.

Uranus in the Sixth House

You like flexibility in your work and day-to-day activities. You do not conform well to routine and are subject to eating unusual foods at weird hours. You like to experiment with different types of diets. You can have unusual illnesses but can also be cured in unorthodox ways. You respond well to cures by electricity, massage, acupuncture, homeopathy, biofeedback, and hypnosis. There could be accidents involving electricity in the workplace and occupational diseases.

Uranus in the Seventh House

You are individualistic and seek others who have unique temperaments. You have an impulsive nature, which can lead to accidents to the ankles or calves. There can be cramping of the lower legs. You can also experience spasmodic kidney pain and lower back spasms. You would benefit from back exercises to relieve tension.

Uranus in the Eighth House

Your life can be exciting, with many ups and downs. There is a need to remain flexible and adaptable, as you are subject to sudden changes. You are prone to spastic conditions of the bowels and need to watch your diet to avoid diseases such as colitis and irritable bowel syndrome. A desire for excitement in the sexual life can lead to venereal diseases.

Uranus in the Ninth House

You follow your own unique philosophy of life. You enjoy traveling to exotic and unusual places, so you should be sure to have the proper inoculations to avoid contracting an unusual disease. You are subject to injury on the lower part of the body while traveling. You need to stretch as often as possible when taking long airplane trips to avoid blood clots and spasms.

Uranus in the Tenth House

You seek the unusual in life, the bizarre and unique. When not allowed to pursue your own course in life, you become tense and nervous and are subject to skin eruptions, stomach upsets, and headaches. There can be joint inflammation and damage to the tendons of the knees as you age. When confronted with a health problem, you would most likely choose an unorthodox method of treatment.

Uranus in the Eleventh House

You have far-reaching goals and enjoy the company of many diverse individuals. You can be nervous and high-strung and need to find ways to relax. There can be accidents to the lower legs, ankles, and calves due to carelessness. You may experience circulatory disorders.

Uranus in the Twelfth House

You have unusual talents and ideas. At times, you lose touch with reality and can become unstable or even paranoid. You can achieve peace of mind through the pursuit of such disciplines as yoga or meditation. You need to be careful in the use of hypnosis, as you may be overly suggestible. You are prone to unusual ailments and need to eat a healthy diet to avoid bowel disorders.

Neptune in the Houses

Neptune in the First House

You can be charismatic, elusive, caring, and romantic. You are sensitive to environmental influences, both mentally and physically. This can involve picking up negativity from persons in your immediate environment as well as being oversensitive to allergens in the environment. Allergic reactions could manifest as skin eruptions on your face. You should have regular eye checkups, as the eyes can be weak. At times, your desire to escape reality can lead to overindulgence in drugs or alcohol.

Neptune in the Second House

You have strong values and can have a nonmaterial attitude toward life. You can be lax in eating habits and indulge yourself in too many sweets. This can cause problems with your blood sugar metabolism, giving the potential for diabetes or hypoglycemia. There can be a weakness in the upper body, which can be strengthened by upper-body exercises. You are also vulnerable to throat infections.

Neptune in the Third House

You are creative and idealistic. You have a weakness in the respiratory system and are prone to respiratory allergies such as hay fever. There are also asthmatic tendencies. You would benefit from breathing exercises to increase lung capacity. You may also be prone to the negative effects of environmental toxins. You should avoid smoking, as the lungs can be weak.

Neptune in the Fourth House

You have a spiritual outlook and may enjoy living near water, which soothes your emotions. You have a sensitive constitution and are prone to food allergies. You may not tolerate dairy products well. The stomach muscles can be weak and would benefit from abdominal exercises.

Neptune in the Fifth House

You are creative and inspired and gain much satisfaction from your creative activities. There is sensitivity in the heart and circulatory areas, and you may benefit from cardiovascular exercises. The middle back can be weak and benefits from stretching and bending exercises. Women with this placement should guard against unwanted pregnancies.

Neptune in the Sixth House

You are a person who derives pleasure from helping others, which aids your emotional well-being. You have a sensitive physique and are subject to infections as well as allergies and overreactions to drugs. You are oversensitive to air pollution, which can affect your breathing. When diagnosed with an illness, you should always get a second opinion, as you can be hard to diagnose. You are prone to peculiar disorders and can have psychosomatic illnesses. You have some tendency toward hypochondria. You may benefit from homeopathic remedies and natural foods.

Neptune in the Seventh House

You are idealistic in relationships and have a romantic view of life. You may overindulge in sweets, which can disturb your blood sugar. You need to drink plenty of water to keep your kidneys flushed, as you are subject to toxic build-up in the kidneys. You may have vitality problems and need to get sufficient rest. The lower back can be weak and benefits from bending and stretching exercises.

Neptune in the Eighth House

You have a mystical outlook on life and enjoy life's mysteries. You may be prone to anemia or other blood ailments and may not adequately process iron. The reproductive and eliminative organs are sensitive. You are prone to infectious diseases such as bladder infections or venereal diseases. Men with this placement can have a weakness in the prostate area. There is a need to eat a healthful diet high in fiber, as there can be weak peristaltic motion in the bowels.

Neptune in the Ninth House

You are a visionary with a strong religious view of life. You need to take the proper precautions when traveling to distant places, as you are prone to infections while traveling. There can be a weakness in the hips and thighs, leading to accidents while traveling. There can be allergic reactions from fumes or gas. You are also prone to edema. You benefit from exercises that build up the lower body.

Neptune in the Tenth House

You are idealistic and can be charismatic and appealing. There can be a weakness in the bones, teeth, and hair, which would benefit from increased minerals in your diet and taking herbs such as silica or horsetail. Toxic substances in the environment can cause a calcium imbalance in your body. You need frequent trips to the dentist, as there is a tendency toward tooth decay. Your knees can be weak, and you may be prone to knee injuries.

Neptune in the Eleventh House

You are idealistic and optimistic about the future. The heart and circulatory systems are vulnerable. Your ankles are weak and can become swollen. There is the danger of sprains. Your circulation can be sluggish and can be helped by exercise such as daily walks.

Neptune in the Twelfth House

You are spiritually oriented and desire a creative life. You are sensitive, both emotionally and physically. You need to build up your immune system, as there can be a proneness to infections or swollen lymph glands. Anxiety can lower your vitality and resistance.

Pluto in the Houses

Pluto in the First House

You have a powerful personality, with a tendency to push yourself to extremes. Throughout your life, you go through periods of elimination and regeneration. There can be radical changes in appearance and the use of cosmetic surgery to alter your appearance. You like to be physically active and also enjoy transforming your body through bodybuilding. You may be prone to endocrine gland malfunctions. There can be hereditary diseases.

Pluto in the Second House

You have a tendency to be rigid and compulsive and need to learn how to relax and let go. You are sensitive to high sugar intake, which can have an adverse effect on health. Your thyroid gland can alternate from hyper to hypo, causing problems in your metabolism. You have a tendency toward infections in the throat area.

Pluto in the Third House

You can be intense and analytical, with a tendency toward compulsive behavior. An overly obsessive nature can put a strain on your nervous system, leading to nervous irritation. The lung area is particularly sensitive and needs to be nourished. There can be a disturbance in the endocrine system, which could be the cause of ailments such as depression.

Pluto in the Fourth House

You have a strong need to feel connected. You feel things intensely and are subject to mood swings, which in turn can affect your energy level. When you are emotionally upset, you may get an upset stomach, indigestion, or in extreme cases an ulcer. Women with this placement may be subject to disorders involving the breasts or womb.

Pluto in the Fifth House

You have an intense nature and natural leadership ability. The heart and circulation are sensitive. You would benefit from some form of cardiovascular exercise to build up your heart. The lower back needs to be guarded in sports, as you are subject to throwing your back out. You have the ability to transform yourself into a healthier individual through diet and exercise.

Pluto in the Sixth House

You can be a tireless worker and are keen and analytical. There is a desire to improve the health throughout your life. The metabolic system as well as the pancreas and intestines are vulnerable with this placement. Your blood sugar metabolism can be out of balance, and you may be prone to diabetes or hypoglycemia. You may benefit from taking pancreatic enzymes. Pluto is associated with enzyme action in the body, and its placement in this house indicates a need for raw foods to aid enzyme action.

Pluto in the Seventh House

You are transformed by relationships and in turn can transform others. You are able to continually reinvigorate your body. You have a weakness in balancing the energies of your body, which can go from one extreme to the other. You need to drink plenty of water every day to keep the kidneys flushed, as you are prone to kidney infections. There can be glandular malfunctions.

Pluto in the Eighth House

You can be intense and powerful. Your relentless drive can put a strain on your nervous system. The reproductive and eliminative organs are sensitive, and too much stress can lead to disorders such as irritable bowel syndrome or colitis. Women with this placement are subject to miscarriage. Men with this placement may have problems with the prostate.

Pluto in the Ninth House

You continually reach out to new horizons and may go through radical changes in outlook. The hips and thighs are sensitive, and it is important to stretch as much as possible on long airplane trips, as there is the potential for sciatica. You have a tendency to overreach and put too much strain on your body as well as to indulge in an unhealthy diet, which puts a strain on the liver. You may be prone to infections while traveling, so you should take proper precautions on any long journey.

Pluto in the Tenth House

You are a born leader with the ability to help others reach their goals. You have much drive and ambition, which can stress your body. You may neglect your health and not eat a balanced diet, which can lead to skin disorders or stomach upsets. Obsessive tendencies can lead to stiff bones and joints and disorders of the knees.

Pluto in the Eleventh House

You are progressive and analytical and a natural group leader. When confronted with a health problem, you like to research and investigate it fully and usually choose alternative health remedies. The heart and circulation are weak areas, and there can be circulatory disorders and stress-related ailments. You tend to run on nervous energy and need to take time out for relaxation.

Pluto in the Twelfth House

You have depth and considerable psychological astuteness. Your immune system is sensitive, and there is proneness to catching colds and flus. You have some tendency to obsess over trivialities or to be in a negative frame of mind. There is a tendency toward morbidity, which can be countered by socializing as much as possible with positive people and engaging in activities you enjoy. Getting involved in the arts and music can lift your spirits.

7
The Health Houses
in Medical Astrology

Chapter 6 provided an overview of all the houses in the chart in terms of medical astrology, as well as interpretations of the planets in the houses. There are two houses in the chart that are traditionally associated with health—the first house, along with the rising sign on the cusp of the first house, known as the Ascendant, and the sixth house, which is known as the house of health. The following will give you a description of your Ascendant along with an interpretation of the planetary aspects made to it, followed by an interpretation of the sign on the cusp of your sixth house of health. (It is necessary to have your exact time of birth to determine an accurate Ascendant.)

The Ascendant and the First House

The Ascendant represents your physical body and appearance. Along with the Sun and Moon in your chart, it is associated with personality characteristics. The sign on your Ascendant, also known as the rising sign, because it is the sign rising on the eastern horizon at the moment of birth, can be a clue to potential health disorders. It can help describe your vitality and physical prowess. It can also describe early environmental influences that may affect health. The sign on the Ascendant can describe how energy is distributed throughout the body and how you resist disease.

The Ascendant is the cusp of the first house. Planets in the first house and planetary aspects to the Ascendant qualify the flow of energy throughout the body. Fire and air signs rising are good conductors of energy. Water and earth signs are more resistant to the flow of energy and need to be stimulated. How others perceive and see you is also described by the Ascendant. These characteristics generally do not refer to health, so they are not part of the following interpretations, which are descriptions of the strengths and weaknesses and potential health disorders associated with each rising sign.

Aries Ascendant

You have a strong physical body and good recuperative powers. You are naturally headstrong and competitive. You tend to be physically active, with strong muscles and much endurance. Exercise is important to you, as it stimulates your natural energy and helps you deal with stress. You can be tireless and tend to push your body too far, which can lead to physical exhaustion or muscle injury. You may experience adrenal exhaustion, which can be helped by vitamin C, parsley, pantothenic acid, vitamin A, zinc, and licorice. You need to guard against accidents to your head and teeth and probably have a facial scar from falling as a child. The head and brain, stomach, and kidneys can be vulnerable areas in your body. You are prone to feverish complaints and skin eruptions on your face caused by an improper diet, allergic reaction, or emotional upset. Men with this placement may become prematurely bald. Nettle and rosemary taken as a tea or used as a rinse can help thinning hair. You may have moles on your face.

Taurus Ascendant

You have a sturdy, muscular, compact body, with much endurance. You can be sensual and pleasure-seeking and are a true gourmet. You are physically strong and may enjoy building up your muscles through weight training. There is also a need to engage in cardiovascular exercise, as you may not be active enough. Your health is good, but you have a tendency toward excess in food, drink, and sex. Being a creature of habit, you tend to eat the same foods and would benefit from eating as varied a diet as possible. A liking for sweets can lead to weight gain or an imbalance in the sugar metabolism in your body. The parts of the body that are sensitive include the throat, thyroid, glands of the neck, ears, jaw, and gums. You are prone to earaches, sore throats, swollen glands, thyroid problems, tonsillitis, gum disease, laryngitis, and a hernia. There is a need for fiber in your diet, as you can be prone to constipation and piles.

Gemini Ascendant

You have a lean physique in a fairly strong body, with good recuperative ability. You are mentally active, very communicative, and like to be on the go. A constant need for mental excitement and a fear of boredom can strain you mentally and physically. You tend to run on nervous energy and need to build up your muscles to increase your physical strength. You are also prone to anxiety and worry, which can lead to nervous irritation. The areas in your body that are vulnerable are the arms, shoulders, lungs, and nervous system. You are prone to respiratory disorders such as asthma, bronchitis, and pneumonia. Smoking is particularly harmful and should be avoided. You are susceptible to accidents in sports that affect the arms, shoulders, and wrists. There can be eyestrain or headaches from mental pressure.

Cancer Ascendant

You have a strong body, which improves with age. You are emotional and sensitive, with a strong need for the bonds of family. Since water signs rising can be somewhat resistant to the flow of energy in the body, you need to engage in a regular schedule of exercise. You are prone to a water imbalance, which can lead to weight gain, and should avoid eating a lot of salty foods that retain water. You have a tendency to overeat when not feeling emotionally satisfied and may have digestive ailments due to overindulgence. You may also experience allergies to milk products. In extreme cases, people with Cancer rising may experience eating disorders such as bulimia or anorexia. The weak points of the body are the chest, breasts, stomach, knees, bones, sinuses, and joints. Emotional distress can lead to ulcers, nausea, or disorders such as gastritis.

Leo Ascendant

You have endurance and vitality and good recuperative powers. You have good powers of resistance, as the vital energies are well distributed in your body. You have a strong sense of pride and dignity, with a craving for attention. You need to feel loved and appreciated to maintain good health. The heart and circulatory system are vulnerable. You are also prone to middle-back ailments, which can be exacerbated by stress. You need to maintain purity of the blood and see to proper elimination to avoid toxins in the blood.

You are a creature of habit, with a tendency to get into ruts at times. You have a liking for rich food, which can raise cholesterol levels in the body. It is important that you engage in an exercise regimen, as you benefit from cardiovascular exercise.

Virgo Ascendant

You have stamina, endurance, and energy. You are analytical and mentally active. Since an earth sign rising can be resistant to the flow of bodily energy, it is important that you are physically active. You are highly intellectual and can have a problem turning off your mind at night. A tendency toward mental upset and worry can result in physical disturbances in the body. You have a sensitive body and need to watch your food intake. People with Virgo rising do well on a diet of natural foods. It is also important that you are watchful of personal hygiene. There is sensitivity in the intestines, liver, and bowels as well as the pancreas. Eating at irregular times or ingesting too many sweets can cause problems with sugar metabolism and the assimilation of vitamins and minerals in your body. It can also result in liver toxicity.

Libra Ascendant

You have good recuperative powers and much vitality. You are friendly and sociable and worry a lot about people liking you. You function best in relationships with others, which are necessary for your emotional well-being. You can become physically ill when in inharmonious situations. Libra is associated with the kidneys and their role in water balance in the body, filtering metabolic waste products from the body, and maintaining the acid/base balance of the blood. Living as rhythmic a life as possible, by eating a balanced diet and avoiding toxic substances, can aid kidney function, which is vulnerable in Libra rising. You are prone to kidney disease, lumbago, and toxins in the blood. There can be an acid/alkaline imbalance in the body. You may crave sweets, which can result in weight gain or a disturbance in the sugar metabolism.

Scorpio Ascendant

You have much endurance, resistance, and muscular strength. You have a strong personality and can be both magnetic and mystifying. You tend to push yourself to extremes, at times being negative and self-destructive in your actions, putting strain and stress on your body. You will experience a lot of psychological changes during your life. Being a person of extremes, you may make abrupt changes in lifestyle and diet, which can lead to problems with the eliminative organs. You have a large appetite with a liking at times for junk food, which can fill your system with toxins. Illness can be severe when it occurs. Like the eliminative system, the reproductive system is also sensitive, and there is a tendency toward sexual excess.

Sagittarius Ascendant

You have vitality, are able to conduct energy throughout your body, and have good recuperative powers. Your positive outlook on life aids your emotional and physical well-being. You always need something to aim for, as a lack of goals or a stagnant existence causes you to become depressed. You can experience mental and nervous strain from not getting enough rest, which can overtax the nervous system. You tend to indulge in high-fat foods, which puts a strain on the liver, a vulnerable part of your body. The weak parts of your body are from the hips to the knees, with a tendency toward ailments such as sciatica. Garlic and iodine are helpful against sciatica. Older persons should protect themselves, as there can be danger of falls and hip injury. A Sagittarius Ascendant also gives a tendency toward feverish ailments and respiratory disorders such as pneumonia, bronchitis, asthma, and pleurisy.

Capricorn Ascendant

You have a strong body constitution and powers of endurance. You are serious-minded, have a strong need for control, and are capable of handling much responsibility. At times, an overly serious attitude can lead to negativity or depression. You may have contracted childhood illnesses, but your physique becomes stronger as you age. It is important that you get plenty of physical exercise to stay limber to aid the flow of energy throughout the body. Capricorn is an earth sign, which can be resistant to the flow of bodily energy. Ailments can affect the skin, bones, and teeth as well as the stomach and breasts. The knees are especially sensitive and should be guarded against accidents. You have a tendency toward falls and bruises, stiff joints, and ailments such as rheumatism and arthritis. People with Capricorn rising need to keep warm, as there can be illness that begins with cold. You are also subject to dental problems if you do not take care of your teeth.

Aquarius Ascendant

You have a strong constitution, vitality, and recuperative powers. As an air sign, Aquarius rising is a good conductor of energy. You are individualistic, eccentric, and unpredictable. Freedom is important to you, and when placed in confining situations, you can feel physically ill. You can be nervous and high-strung, with a tendency to overreact emotionally, and can experience tics or spasms. You can wear yourself out from nervous excitement and need periods of calm to regain vitality. There is a vulnerability in the calves and ankles and a tendency toward circulatory disorders, sprained or broken legs or ankles, and nervous disorders. You can have a problem with cold extremities. You are subject to unusual illnesses. You thrive on fresh air and would do well in the mountains.

Pisces Ascendant

Your vitality is uneven but is helped by rest. Water signs rising can be resistant to the flow of bodily energies and need stimulation from food or exercise. You are idealistic and sensitive and can be a visionary. Spiritual and creative activities soothe your emotions and aid your health. You do not handle stress well and sometimes overindulge in alcohol or drugs to relieve stress. You are prone to anxiety and mental strain, which can lower resistance and lead to illness. Your immune system is highly sensitive and needs to be built up. Also sensitive are the liver and bowels. You need to keep your digestive organs and bowels in good condition through diet. Your feet are also sensitive, and there can be toe and foot problems such as corns, bunions, or athlete's foot. As a water sign rising, there is a tendency toward flabbiness, and you need exercise to avoid becoming overweight in middle age.

Planetary Aspects to the Ascendant

The following is a list of planetary aspects to the Ascendant with a description of their effects on health. The aspects are categorized as favorable (sextile, trine) or stressful (square, opposition).

To interpret a conjunction to the Ascendant, please refer to "The Planets in the Houses in Medical Astrology" in chapter 6. If you have a planet rising in your chart, you can consider it to be conjunct the Ascendant, and can use the definition given for that planet in the first house for an explanation of the meaning. For example, if you have the Mars conjunct your Ascendant (rising in your chart), you would read the description of Mars in the first house.

A planet conjunct the Ascendant is more powerful than when the planet just occupies the first house, but the basic meaning is the same. A planet conjunct the Ascendant can also alter the interpretation of the Ascendant.

Sun Sextile/Trine the Ascendant

You have a strong constitution, with much vitality and endurance. You have a strong personality and are vibrant and outgoing. Your enjoyment of physical activity is an aid to good health. You have excellent powers of resistance.

Sun Square/Opposition the Ascendant

You have the same attributes as the Sun sextile/trine the Ascendant, but some tendency to push yourself too hard, leading to vitality problems. When ill, you tend toward feverish or inflammatory complaints. Illness can begin with cold. You can have personality conflicts due to an overwhelming need for attention. Your eyes are also sensitive, and you benefit from regular eye checkups.

Moon Sextile/Trine the Ascendant

This is a beneficial contact that adds vitality and benefits the emotional nature. There is strong resistance to disease and the ability to overcome fatigue and maintain a steady energy level. This aspect aids the personality, as you are easy to get along with and helpful to others.

Moon Square/Opposition the Ascendant

There is an inconstancy to your personality and an uneven flow of energy throughout your body. You are subject to disorders caused by stress and by poor eating habits and health routines. Your mood swings can prove disconcerting to others. You are emotionally vulnerable, can be overly subjective, and need to learn to be more objective and less subject to the whims of your emotions. There can be a water imbalance in the body, and you are subject to sudden weight gain and loss. You may have unusual food cravings. Your body is overly sensitive, and you are subject to allergic reactions. Women with this position may experience PMS.

Mercury Sextile/Trine the Ascendant

You are mobile and active and very communicative. You have energy and vitality and good powers of recuperation. You thrive on being busy. You have a sound nervous system and mental stability.

Mercury Square/Opposition the Ascendant

You have vitality and energy but tend to run on nervous energy, which can lead to frayed nerves and nervous irritability. You have a tendency to worry and are prone to anxiety. There can be nervous and respiratory disorders as well as a hormonal imbalance. In extreme instances, there is mental imbalance or mental illness.

Venus Sextile/Trine the Ascendant

You are kind and generous and have a pleasant personality. You are sociable and thrive on social outings and the pursuit of pleasure. You seek enjoyment and comfort and can feel ill in disharmonious surroundings. You may have a sweet tooth, which can lead to weight gain or dental problems.

Venus Square/Opposition the Ascendant

You can be lazy and self-indulgent. You enjoy sweets and tend to overindulge in food and drink, which can lead to disorders caused by excess. There is a vulnerability in the throat and kidneys, and you are prone to ailments such as swollen glands, sore throat, and kidney disease.

Mars Sextile/Trine the Ascendant

You have much vitality and physical endurance. You have sound muscles and enjoy physical activity. You have healthy blood and resistance to infection. You have the ability to bounce back quickly from illness. A love of activity keeps you healthy.

Mars Square/Opposition the Ascendant

You have similar attributes to Mars sextile/trine the Ascendant, but you can be more aggressive and competitive, with an impulsive nature that can make you accident-prone. You love speed and find it hard to slow down, leading to physical exhaustion or burnout. There is also the potential for blood disorders such as anemia. There can be adrenal burnout. When ill, there can be fever and inflammatory disorders as well as the potential for cuts, bruises, and scalds. There can be muscular disorders and infections. There is the potential for surgery at some time in the life.

Jupiter Sextile/Trine the Ascendant

This position confers vitality and optimism. Your hopeful outlook on life is an aid to good health. There is the ability to bounce back from disease. You benefit from outdoor exercise and sports activity.

Jupiter Square/Opposition the Ascendant

This aspect has many of the positive attributes of Jupiter sextile/trine the Ascendant, but there is a tendency toward exaggeration and a lack of moderation. A liking for rich foods can lead to weight gain and put a strain on the liver. There can be blood disorders and illness resulting from overeating or overindulgence.

Saturn Sextile/Trine the Ascendant

You have endurance, vitality, and good resistance to disease. You thrive on hard work and have a sound bone structure. You tend toward moderation in food and drink, which is an aid to longevity.

Saturn Square/Opposition the Ascendant

You may have vitality problems and a hindered flow of energy, with lowered resistance. There can be hereditary diseases and illness in early childhood. It is important to eat foods high in minerals, as there can be a weakness in the bones and teeth. You are subject to ear problems and could experience a loss of hearing in your later years. You may have a chronic disease as well as skin troubles. It is important to avoid getting chilled in cold weather, as illness can arise from cold. Diet is especially important, as you can be undernourished or not assimilate vitamins and minerals properly. An overly somber attitude can lead to depression and a lowering of vitality.

Uranus Sextile/Trine the Ascendant

You are bright, intuitive, and intelligent. You keep up with the latest information on diet and nutrition and are willing to try a new fitness regimen if you think it will improve your health. Engaging in outdoor exercise aids your circulatory system and oxygenation processes in the body, keeping you vital and alert. You benefit from breathing exercises and fresh air.

Uranus Square/Opposition the Ascendant

You have similar characteristics to Uranus sextile/trine the Ascendant, but are more prone to tension-related ailments due to an inability to relax. There is an uneven flow of energy throughout your body, which is alleviated by exercise or meditation. You do not handle stress well and need to find a way to release tension through leisure activities. You are vulnerable to high blood pressure, nervous complaints, cramps, nervous strain, accidents, trigeminal neuralgia, circulatory complaints, headaches, and tension-related ailments.

Neptune Sextile/Trine the Ascendant

You are sensitive and compassionate and could be considered a visionary. You find serenity through contact with water and can be rejuvenated by sea air. You spiritual nature is an aid to emotional balance.

Neptune Square/Opposition the Ascendant

You have changing energy patterns and vitality leaks. You need to eat a nutritious diet and live in a healthy environment, as a polluted atmosphere has a negative effect on your physical well-being. You have a desire to escape reality and can become addicted to drugs or alcohol. You are overly sensitive to drugs and may need lower doses of prescribed medicines. You should always get a second opinion on any medical diagnosis, as there can be misdiagnoses, masked symptoms, or misread lab tests. There can be lowered immunity, resulting in colds and flus. You are hypersensitive and prone to allergies. Illness can result from drugs or poisons. You are also prone to viruses, parasites, and fungus infections. There can be poor muscle tone due to a lack of exercise.

Pluto Sextile/Trine the Ascendant

You have tremendous vitality and recuperative powers. You have the energy to surmount illness and transform your body in a healthy manner. You have a powerful personality and leadership ability. You have stamina and psychological astuteness. You have the ability to eliminate toxins from your body.

Pluto Square/Opposition the Ascendant

You have the attributes of Pluto sextile/trine the Ascendant, but you have a tendency to push your body to its limits. You are prone to inflammatory or infectious disorders and abscesses. There can also be skin disorders. There can be hereditary disorders and disorders of the endocrine glands. You can react negatively in the form of an allergic reaction to the effects of toxins in the environment.

The Sixth House in Medical Astrology

The sixth house has traditionally been called the house of health. It can describe your daily routines and habits, and their effects on your health. One can derive diet and nutritional information from the sixth house, as it is a house of assimilation and nutrition. It is linked with work and can describe work-related ailments, including stress-related or industrial diseases. Through an analysis of this house, one may observe energy fluctuations, the work environment, and the type of work you perform.

The sixth house describes how one's work affects health in such matters as repetitive types of jobs that could cause injury to the hands or wrists; jobs involving machinery that could lead to an accident; jobs in an unhealthy environment or that utilize chemicals that can lead to allergies or other toxic disorders; and jobs causing conflicts with coworkers, leading to mental stress or depression. Needless to say, unfulfilling work or overwork can also lead to mental stress or depression. One can understand health habits and observe the sign on the cusp of the sixth house and planets therein as a guide to specific disease states. People who are happy in their work tend to be optimistic, which is an aid to well-being. One may also observe inherited genetic patterns in this house.

To interpret your sixth house, first read the meaning of the sign on the cusp from the following list of descriptions. If you have any planets in your sixth house, refer to "The Planets in the Houses in Medical Astrology" in chapter 6 for an interpretation of a specific planet in the sixth house. More advanced astrology students may want to study the planet ruling the cusp of their sixth house. If the ruler of your sixth house receives many stressful aspects, it could indicate that you have poor health habits. (See chapter 3 for an interpretation of a planet in terms of health.)

Aries on the Cusp of the Sixth House

This position can indicate a high energy level and a vibrant state of health. The circulation is good, with a rich blood supply. You need plenty of exercise, which feeds both your vascular system and your nervous system. You prefer work that utilizes a lot of energy and may enjoy competing with co-workers. You would not do well in a sedentary job, as you are naturally active and can actually feel ill when confined for a long period of time. You need to be on the go as much as possible to ensure a healthy outlook on life. This position can indicate the potential for accidents at work due to carelessness or impulsive behavior. Use care around machinery and sharp objects. There is also the potential for burnout, as Aries rule the adrenals and overexertion without rest can lead to adrenal exhaustion. Ailments affect the head and eyes and can be expressed as headaches, head injuries, dental problems, or sinus problems. Mars rules Aries, and its position and aspects should be examined.

Taurus on the Cusp of the Sixth House

This position gives resistance and endurance. You enjoy working in peaceful surroundings, possibly doing something related to the arts or beauty. You like comfortable surroundings with congenial people and dislike moving around a lot. You require security in work, as job insecurity can cause stress, which could upset your sugar metabolism. Illness can be chronic and severe when it does occur, and a big appetite can strain the heart and put toxins in your system. Ailments affect the throat, neck, ears, tonsils, vocal cords, and esophagus. Venus rules Taurus, and its position and aspects should be examined.

Gemini on the Cusp of the Sixth House

This position gives energy and vitality. There can be a desire to work in occupations that require the use of the mind and are intellectually stimulating, as you can easily become bored. If involved in work you dislike, there can be depression and anxiety. You have the ability to engage in more than one activity at a time. You are good with your hands and need to guard against work-related injuries to the arms and hands. You are also susceptible to airborne pollutants in the workplace, which can lead to respiratory problems such as bronchitis or asthma or allergic reactions. Proper breathing is important for maintenance of health. You are susceptible to lung ailments as well as to fractures of the arms or wrists. Your nervous system is also sensitive, and you are subject to nervous disorders when in a difficult work situation. You do not handle stress well. Mercury rules Gemini, and its position and aspects should be examined.

Cancer on the Cusp of the Sixth House

Your emotions greatly affect your health. When you feel in control and enjoy your work, your health prospers. You enjoy work that allows you to nurture others and work at your own pace. When forced to do work you dislike, ailments can arise in the stomach, abdominal region, breasts, sternum, or ribs. Ailments range from stomach upset, nausea, and flatulence to severe gastric distress. You are prone to stomach allergies, possibly from seafood. You can also be prone to emotional disorders such as worry and anxiety. Above all, you need to find work that is emotionally satisfying to stay healthy. The Moon rules Cancer, and its position and aspects should be examined.

Leo on the Cusp of the Sixth House

You generally have good health and are able to surmount illness quickly. The heart as well as the spine and back are vulnerable with this placement, and there can be a genetic heart weakness in your family. You are a person who needs to have some control or authority over what you do for a living. You are happiest in work that allows your creative juices to flow, and you enjoy being the center of attention. When feeling stressed from work, there can be problems with the middle back. You would benefit from eating a heart-healthy diet and from doing exercises that help your back remain supple. The Sun rules Leo, and its position and aspects should be examined.

Virgo on the Cusp of the Sixth House

You have the sign of work on the cusp of the house of work (and health). You can be a tireless worker and need to work to feel emotionally stable. You don't mind drudgery in work and are pleased to be able to be of service to others. Overwork can put a strain on your nervous system, which is vulnerable with this placement. As this is also the natural house of diet, maintaining good health depends on keeping the digestive organs and bowels in good working order. Virgo rules discrimination and assimilation, and you tend to have good instincts for the right foods. You may experience allergies to products containing wheat. The pancreas is ruled by Virgo, which can be aided by pancreatic enzymes. Mercury rules Virgo, and its position and aspects should be examined.

Libra on the Cusp of the Sixth House

You have an innate sense of beauty, which can be used in professions involving the arts. You are also adept in human relations and would enjoy work that allows you to use your diplomatic skills. You can feel unwell in inharmonious working conditions and would dislike working in any place that seems sterile and lacks beauty. You find disharmonious relations with co-workers particularly upsetting, and could develop skin eruptions as a result. The kidneys are also vulnerable with this position, as is the lower back. Disharmonious working conditions could result in lower back pain. Venus rules Libra, and its position and aspects should be examined.

Scorpio on the Cusp of the Sixth House

This combination gives good endurance. You desire work that allows you to be in charge or that has depth, such as research or investigation. You do not submit well to others giving you orders, and if put in this position, you could develop bowel disorders. The throat and the reproductive and eliminative organs are sensitive with this placement. This position can also indicate someone working in a healing profession. The more you are able to heal others, the greater strength you feel, which is an aid to good health. Pluto rules Scorpio, and its position and aspects should be examined.

Sagittarius on the Cusp of the Sixth House

You have vitality and good recuperative powers, but mental stress and a nervous disposition can put a strain on your health. You need to be in a job that provides the opportunity for growth. You like to be mentally stimulated in your work. You dislike working in a closed-in environment. Outdoor work such as ranching or work that allows you to be on the go would appeal to you. You are prone to accidents at work that affect the hips or thighs. Also vulnerable are your lungs, which could be adversely affected by working in industries that produce industrial waste or utilize chemicals. You are also susceptible to blood impurities, which manifest as boils and abscesses. You are prone to accidents resulting from travel, sports, or animals. Jupiter rules Sagittarius, and its position and aspects should be examined.

Capricorn on the Cusp of the Sixth House

This is a placement that gets better with age. You are responsible and disciplined and need work that allows you some measure of authority and control. When ill, you may experience aches and pains, especially in the joints. You are also prone to colds, chills, digestive ailments, falls, and skin ailments. You may experience uneven energy levels, which can be helped by diet and exercise. You can be a strict disciplinarian and are able to follow a special diet when necessary. Capricorn is ruled by Saturn, and its position and aspects should be examined.

Aquarius on the Cusp of the Sixth House

You have a sound body and good mental powers. You need work that allows you to be inventive and gives you freedom of action. You don't mind working irregular hours and prefer to work at your own pace. You also may eat at irregular hours, causing your body to be off-rhythm. This can lead to nervousness or nervous disorders. Ailments can affect the circulatory system, the ankles, and the electrical system of the body. There is a need for quiet times to recharge your nervous system. You also like to try the latest health fad and are attracted to new age cures rather than traditional medicine. Aquarius is ruled by Uranus, and its position and aspects should be examined.

Pisces on the Cusp of the Sixth House

You are sensitive and intuitive and require work that gives you inspiration. Work involving fantasy, such as film, or that lets you use your imagination appeals to you. You become easily depressed when involved in work that is uncreative or uninspiring. Your immune system is sensitive, and you may be prone to colds or flus, mucous conditions, and respiratory disorders. The liver is also a sensitive area, and it is important that you eat a healthy diet and avoid fried foods. You need to take care of your feet, which are prone to problems such as corns or bunions. Neptune rules Pisces, and its position and aspects should be examined.

8
The Elements in Medical Astrology

The four elements—fire, earth, air, and water—can help you pinpoint some obvious and easy-to-correct factors that affect health. Too much or not enough of an element can contribute to weaknesses in various parts of the body. By compensating for a lack of or an emphasis in an element, one can alter the imbalance and improve health.

Excess Fire

In medical astrology, the fire element refers to physical energy and the digestive processes. Excess fire in the chart generates a lot of body heat. Your physical energy is high, and there is a potential to burn yourself out, leading to exhaustion and adrenal burnout. You need to learn how to conserve your physical energy. Your tendency to push yourself to your limits puts a lot of wear and tear on your physical body. This continual stress on the body can lead to conditions such as high blood pressure, migraines, or ulcers. You may also be prone to excess perspiration and become easily dehydrated, so you need to replenish fluids frequently in your body. You may be hot-tempered and angry. You can be pushy and egocentric, thinking only of your own needs. You can be highly impatient, with a tendency toward heartburn, liver problems, and stomach and gallbladder disorders.

People with excess fire need to limit their consumption of spices and stimulants. You need to balance your fiery nature by consuming foods that are cold or moist. You would benefit from bland foods such as raw or steamed vegetables, juicy fruits, and dairy products, as well as relaxation techniques such as yoga and meditation. A cold shower or water activities such as swimming or sailing can calm the fiery energies. Spices such as cumin, coriander, fennel, and dill are good for fiery types. Artistic activity could also be used as an outlet.

Low Fire

Low fire in the chart can have adverse effects on both your mental and physical health. You can be lethargic, lack courage, and have a lack of confidence, leading to poor self-esteem. You may experience vitality problems and have poor digestion. You may have poor circulation, poor muscle tone, and indigestion. There can be a lack of energy to resist disease. Body heat is low, and you may be subject to sluggishness and depression. The liver and gallbladder may not be working up to par.

There are various ways to increase the fire element. Engaging in some type of physical exercise on a regular basis can increase the fire element. Gradually adding more spices and sour foods to your diet can stimulate digestion as well as the absorption of nutrients. Foods such as lemons and yogurt and spices such as cayenne, cinnamon, cardamom, curry, ginger, or peppermint tea can aid the digestion. You can bring the element of fire into your life by utilizing the colors red and orange in your clothing and decor. Herbs that stimulate the liver and gallbladder, such as burdock root or dandelion leaf, may be taken. Lighting candles or using a fireplace increases the fire element. Aerobic-type exercises will strengthen the heart and circulatory system. Singular activities that increase self-confidence, such as rollerskating, ice skating, skiing, hiking, or mountain climbing, will increase the fire element.

Excess Earth

Excess earth in the chart can cause a feeling of sluggishness in the body and a sense of lethargy. There is a tendency for a stocky or overweight body. You probably don't exercise enough. You can be rigid and compulsive and can be overly obsessed with your body. Your metabolism can be slow. Healthwise, you may experience deposits in the joints and arteries and develop health problems due to an imbalance of heavy metals and calcium.

The body can experience blockages and physical congestion. You need to stimulate your digestion, which is sluggish. This can be done by eating foods containing spices such as cayenne and ginger, getting more exercise, and eating light foods such as fruit salads, sprouts, and vegetables. Cut down on heavy foods, such as meat and potatoes, that require a long time to digest. You need to drink plenty of water and limit your consumption of dairy products. Avoid eating in between meals, as you need to allow plenty of time for food to digest. Utilizing bright yellow and orange in your decor can help energize excess earth. Engaging in some type of precision sport, such as pool, tennis, golf, or badminton, can help increase agility and overcome the sluggishness of earth.

Low Earth

With a chart low in earth, you can appear to be spacey, dreamy, or unstable. You can be unrealistic or impractical, and you do not manage your time well. Others may see you as unreliable. There is a need to deal with the tangible, practical world.

You can be out of touch with the needs of your body and ignore warning signals of a potential health disorder. You may eat on the run or skip meals. You do not always get enough outdoor exercise or sunlight. You may have poor skin tone. There can be bone weakness, which is helped by exercise and a diet containing sufficient vitamins and minerals. You can be helped by grounding techniques such as a regular schedule of eating, sleeping, and relaxing. Other grounding techniques include gardening or communing more with nature, perhaps by taking a trip to a national park or driving through the countryside. You can increase the earth element by wearing earth colors such as browns and greens, having plants in the house, and spending more time outdoors. A weekly massage can also increase your body awareness.

Eating heavy foods can ground you. These include root vegetables, such as carrots, potatoes, turnips, beets, and squash. You can also benefit by including whole grains, brown rice, nuts, oils, cheese, butter, garlic, onions, and spices such as ginger and curry in your diet. Ginseng, pineapple, and fennel can be helpful in stimulating digestion.

Excess Air

The air element refers to the circulation of the body, the nervous system, respiration, and communication. With an excess of air in the chart, you are highly intelligent but can be detached and impersonal. You tend to ignore the needs of the body, as you are good at rationalizing. You have an overactive mind, which can lead to nervous exhaustion. Your nervous system is highly charged and extremely sensitive. You tend to be nervous, jittery, and anxious. You appear to be energetic but tend to run on nervous energy, without having any real stamina. There is a strong mental component with excess air, with an inability to turn off the mind, leading to insomnia. Teas such as chamomile, skullcap, vervain, and valerian can help calm the nerves. Activities such as yoga or breathing exercises can aid the nervous system. There can be tics and spasms caused by an overload on the nervous system. You need periods of rest and relaxation to allow the nervous system to recharge itself.

You are prone to ailments such as asthma, anemia, flatulence, and muscle spasms and pain. Peppermint tea can help both muscle spasms and digestive disorders. You may be prone to headaches and indigestion. Excess air dries up water, which can lead to thirst and dehydration. You tend toward dryness, causing dry, rough skin, brittle hair and nails, stiff joints, and diseases such as arthritis. You need to increase your intake of fluids, especially water. You benefit from eating whole grains and taking B-complex vitamins and magnesium.

Low Air

With a deficiency of air in the chart, you may have poor communication skills and a dislike of socializing. You can lack a sense of humor. You need to think things through more carefully before making an important decision. You may have a difficulty in the flow of bodily energies, leading to poor circulation, a weak nervous system, tiredness, shortness of breath, and slowness of movement. Your body can lack elasticity and flexibility. Movement such as dancing and yoga can increase flexibility. Low air can be helped by deep-breathing exercises and fresh, circulating air. A trip to the mountains can be rejuvenating. Wearing sky colors such as blue and coral can help. Pleasant sounds such as music can be calming and increase the air element. Heavy foods should be kept to a minimum, as they add to the heaviness of having low air. Eat plenty of raw fruits and vegetables. Juices, sprouts, and grains should be added to the diet.

Excess Water

With an excess of water in the chart, you can appear to others as dreamy and spacey. You are highly emotional and can become defensive at times. You are prone to depression and moodiness. You need to learn detachment. You need to use psychic self-defense to avoid picking up negative vibrations around you. You can learn to channel your emotions in a positive way by getting involved in a creative project. Because water is cold, wet, and heavy, an excess can contribute to phlegm and mucus discharges in the body, which affect the lungs and throat. You may be prone to colds and lymphatic congestion. Excess water aids in eliminating toxins from the body, but you can become waterlogged and overweight. You are prone to diseases involving discharges or a build-up of fluids in the body. You can be overly sensitive to pollutants in the air, leading to allergies. You would benefit from living by the sea and breathing salt air and exercising more.

People with excess water benefit from ingesting bitter herbs and utilizing diuretic herbs such as dandelion leaf, nettles, and alfalfa. The consumption of sweets and dairy products should be kept low. Foods that retain water, such as bread and salt and especially melons, should also be kept to a minimum. The heaviness of water needs to be balanced by lighter foods such as dried fruits and salads and hot spices such as cayenne and ginger. Eating brittle foods that crumble, such as crackers and chips, helps reduce excess water. Exercise is also beneficial.

Low Water

With a deficiency of water in the chart, you tend to be restless, jittery, anxious, unstable at times, and fearful. You may have difficulty understanding your own emotions, and you can lack empathy. You can have problems showing emotions. Blocked emotions can lead to physical problems in the body that can cause an energy blockage. There can also be water blockages in the body and poor or slow healing.

Hair, bones, and nails can be brittle, and you may have stiff joints and dry skin. You may be thirsty all the time and have to be careful of dehydration. There can be a difficulty in eliminating toxins from the body, which can be helped by drinking plenty of fluids every day. You benefit from drinking fresh spring water.

You need foods that are rich, oily, and moist and can benefit from herbs that absorb moisture, such as Iris moss, slippery elm, and licorice. Diuretic herbs should be used with care. You should eat lots of juicy fruits and vegetables, drink vegetable juices, and include more soup in your diet. Limit your consumption of raw diuretic vegetables, such as carrots, celery, cabbage, and asparagus. Salt is acceptable but not in large quantities.

Having an aquarium, joining a pool club, taking baths instead of showers, using bath oils, going to a sauna, going scuba diving, or swimming all increase the water element. Living near water increases the water element. An interest in the arts can also increase the water element.

9
The Modes in Medical Astrology

The modes consist of the three types of energy displayed by the signs of the zodiac. The modes, also known as modalities or qualities, are defined as cardinal, fixed, or mutable. They are also referred to as the cardinal, fixed, or mutable crosses. They provide the astrologer with a form of classification of the signs of the zodiac. The cardinal signs are Aries, Cancer, Libra, and Capricorn; the fixed signs are Taurus, Leo, Scorpio, and Aquarius; and the mutable signs are Gemini, Virgo, Sagittarius, and Pisces.

In medical astrology, illness is classified as either a cardinal type of illness, a fixed type of illness, or a mutable type of illness. The following descriptions of the modes describe each type.

Cardinal Mode

With an emphasis of planets in the cardinal signs in the chart, you can be demanding and willful. You are a troubleshooter, you like to be in on the action, and you have a strong need to succeed. You like to solve problems through direct action. In fact, you propel yourself through life with such energy that you may overwhelm others, causing them to react in a negative manner toward you. People born with a cardinal emphasis in their chart tend to rush headlong into situations, often without thinking, and may try to push themselves beyond the limits of the body. There is a need to learn to recognize your own limits and a need for self-discipline and self-control.

You can benefit from the use of meditation and quiet periods of reflection. Physical disciplines such as yoga and tai chi are also beneficial. An excessive amount of cardinal energy can describe type-A behavior. There is a need to slow down.

The parts of the body that can be affected when you have a majority of planets in cardinal signs include the chest area, stomach, rib cage, head, kidneys, bones, and gallbladder. You may find that some of your health problems are due to a weakness in the kidneys or gallbladder. Illness tends to be acute. When you do have a health problem, you are not afraid to try new treatments or medications. You are also impatient for results.

Fixed Mode

With a majority a planets in the fixed signs in the chart, you are reliable, but you can be stubborn and rigid and resistant to change. A lack of flexibility causes you to get stuck in a rut. An overly stiff demeanor can manifest as stiffness in the body. Fixed-type illnesses can be cumulative in nature, resulting in growths, cysts, blockages, or enlargement of a body part. There can be a sluggishness to the body that can be helped by increased physical exercise. You need variety in your diet and plenty of roughage. You would also benefit from body therapies such as rolfing and bioenergetics. Fixed-type diseases are chronic and can last a long time. It can be a disorder you live with much of your life. The parts of the body affected include the throat, reproductive and eliminative organs, heart, and circulatory system. Fixed-cross problems may be related to problems with the colon or thyroid gland. A diet high in liquids, juices, fruits, and vegetables is helpful. Consumption of heavy foods should be restricted.

Mutable Mode

With a majority of planets in the mutable signs in the chart, you are flexible and adaptable but have a tendency to scatter your energies. You are people-oriented and need a lot of mental stimulation. At times you become hyper and experience insomnia from trying to do too much at once. Many of your problems stem from an inability to relax or concentrate. You are easily distracted and are prone to anxiety or worry. There can be a mental component to your illnesses. You have some tendency toward hypochondria. Learning to finish one thing at a time before starting a new project will help calm your nervous system.

You are prone to diseases that affect the lungs, intestines, nervous system, and immune system. You are subject to sudden illness but usually have a quick recovery. However, there can be recurring illnesses. You may find that the cause of your illnesses relates to the lymph glands or pancreas. You need to build up your immune system and watch your sugar intake. Foods containing vitamins A, B, and C and zinc aid the immune system. There can be metabolic disorders due to improper glucose production. There can also be illnesses difficult to treat such as hypertension, ulcers, and headaches. You can benefit from meditation, biofeedback, or acupuncture. You need time to relax. Grounding techniques, such as gardening or communing with nature, or disciplines that focus the attention, such as yoga and tai chi, are beneficial.

Appendix A
Nutritional Guidance to Nourish Weak Areas of the Body

The following list includes remedies to help build up weak areas of the body as well as aid various disorders. It does not purport to be complete but includes helpful herbs and foods as well as information on vitamins and minerals for various disorders of the body. One should see a doctor or a nutritionist to get a full understanding of any health disorder.

Acid Conditions: Blueberries, huckleberries, alfalfa, celery, peppermint tea, magnesium.

Acne: Aloe vera, zinc, vitamin B6, vitamin A, red clover tea.

Adrenals: Vitamin C, parsley, pantothenic acid, vitamin A, zinc, licorice, ginseng.

Alkalinity: Oranges.

Allergies: A juice made from carrots, cucumber, and celery aid mucous membranes. Also, vitamins A, B, C, and E, bioflavonoids, magnesium, red clover tea, rosehips tea, echinacea root.

Anemia: Apricots, plums, raisins, black currants, strawberries, bananas, beets, broccoli, carrots, cherries, lentils, radishes, spinach, tomatoes, sunflower seeds, unsulphured blackstrap molasses, liver, meat, beans, dried fruit, whole grain products, beet greens, eggs, kefir, vitamin C, cobalt, copper, calcium, folic acid, niacin, vitamin B6, bee pollen.

Arteries: Calcium, copper, vitamin B, natural oils; also, a carrots, garlic, and pineapple juice combination. Cut out foods such as doughnuts and potato chips.

Arteriosclerosis: Liquid chlorophyll, vitamin B, potassium, calcium, vitamin D, garlic.

Arthritis: Cherries, celery, fresh fruit and vegetable juices, parsley, alfalfa, watercress, kelp, seaweed, raw celery, grapefruit, apples, carrots, magnesium, red clover tea, goldenseal tea, skullcap tea, kelp.

Asthma: Comfrey tea,[1] fenugreek tea, aloe vera, vitamin E, white turnip juice, thyme, caraway, vitamin E, potassium, acupuncture.

Bladder: Iron, magnesium, vitamin A, vitamin D, manganese, potassium, parsley tea, corn silk tea, strawberry leaf tea, juniper berry tea, asparagus.

Bladder Infection: Fresh cranberries, pomegranate, yogurt, buttermilk, uva ursi, buchu.

Blood: Strawberry leaf tea, red clover tea, comfrey tea,[2] borage tea, hyssop tea, yarrow tea, dandelion, aloe vera, wheatgrass, raw carrots, beets, black currants, raspberries, lemons, blackberries, blueberries, casaba melon, pineapple, watercress, watermelon, sunflower seeds, carrot juice, citrus fruits.

Bones: Magnesium, vitamin D, vitamin C, calcium, silicon, brown rice, goat cheese, Roquefort cheese, whole wheat, corn, kale.

Bowels: Fruit with fiber, spinach, alfalfa sprouts, peaches, plums, prunes, squash, bananas.

Brain: Phosphorus, potassium, vitamins B, C, and E, vanadium, magnesium, lettuce, citrus fruits, olive oil, nut oils, beef, corn, smoked halibut, walnuts, almonds, limes, sea bass.

Breasts: Kelp, magnesium, yarrow tea.

Breathing: Vitamin C, vitamin A.

Bronchitis: Vitamin A, vitamin D, calcium, iron, chlorine, phosphorus, garlic, sunflower seeds, caraway, fenugreek tea, clove oil, white onions, white turnip juice.

Calcification (of Tissues): Vitamins A, B, C, D, and E, calcium, phosphorus, yogurt, wheatgrass.

Candida Albicans (Yeast Infection): Avoid yeast, refined sugars, vinegars, mushrooms, aged cheese, dried fruits, fruit juices. Eat yogurt containing live acidophilus cultures.

Cardiovascular Disease: Cut down on meats. Eat more legumes. Avoid high-fat foods. Include one or more tablespoons of olive oil in your diet each day. Watch your cholesterol levels. Snack on unsalted sunflower or pumpkin seeds. Bananas, potatoes, asparagus, buckwheat, and millet are good for you. Increase omega-3 fatty acids, calcium, carnitine, and magnesium. Include onions and garlic in your diet. Also, wheat germ, borage tea, manganese, lecithin, pectin, chromium, vitamin B1, vitamin B6, niacin, folic acid, vitamin C, selenium, vitamin E, fish, hawthorn tea.

Carpal Tunnel Syndrome: Vitamin B6.

Catarrh: Vitamin A, magnesium, iodine, raw pineapple, raw garlic, wintergreen, fenugreek tea, horehound tea, comfrey tea,[3] red radishes, lemons, leeks, apricots, cherries, grapefruit, white onions, oranges, pineapple.

Cholesterol-Lowering Foods: Lecithin, olive oil, canola oil, garlic, avocados, onions, dietary fiber, soy, alfalfa, artichokes, cabbage, eggplant, fenugreek tea, skullcap tea.

Circulatory Problems: Vitamin E, niacin, bioflavonoids, zinc.

Colitis: Vitamin A, lecithin, vitamin B-complex, digestive enzymes, avocados, tapioca. Avoid cabbage, cucumber, grapefruit.

Colon: Spinach juice, vitamin A, comfrey,[4] lecithin.

Constipation: Raw spinach, apple juice, apples, carrots, pumpkin seeds, yogurt, eggplant, black figs, pineapple, soaked dried fruits, unpeeled apples, melon, psyllium seed tea, catnip tea, sennapod tea before retiring, magnesium, vitamin B-complex, flaxseed.

Cough: Licorice root boiled in water, fenugreek tea, comfrey.[5]

Cystitis: Vitamin A, vitamin C, goldenseal root tea, licorice root tea, uva ursi, buchu, juniper berries.

Diabetes Mellitus: Eat sensibly. Cut down on alcohol and tobacco. Herbs: horsetail, dandelion, licorice root, alfalfa, and Oregon grape root. Also, chromium, zinc, vitamin C, foods containing potassium, blueberries, huckleberries, string beans, Brussels sprouts, raw fresh vegetables, brewer's yeast, wheat grass, lentils, parsley.

Diarrhea: Vitamin A, raw garlic, pumpkin seeds, peppermint tea, raw pulped apple.

Digestion: Ginseng, beet tops, kefir, fennel, pineapple, yogurt, kiwi fruit, mugwort, mint tea.

Digestive Disorders: Avoid spicy foods. Add fiber to your diet. Eat more salads. Also, pineapples, bananas, dates.

Diuretic: Celery, watermelon, juniper berries, horsetail, watercress.

Diverticulitis: Aloe vera, comfrey,[6] oranges.

Earache: Hops, pumpkin.

Eczema: Aloe vera gel, comfrey tea,[7] sunflower seeds, strawberry leaf tea.

Edema: Caused by a deficiency of magnesium and sodium. Helped by vitamin B6, potassium, watermelon seeds, pumpkin seeds, squash seeds.

Endocrine Glands: Ginseng, greens, silicon, sodium, vitamins A, B, C, and E, iodine, calcium, phosphorous, lecithin, organic fluorine.

Eyes: B vitamins especially riboflavin, vitamins A, C, and D, calcium, chlorophyll, zinc, fennel, carrots, parsley, celery, kefir, almonds, asparagus, broccoli, liver, wheat germ, butter, eyebright tea.

Fatigue: Ginseng root, gotu kola (a Chinese herb), licorice root, cayenne, garlic, magnesium, vitamins A, B, C, and D, iron, iodine, potassium, manganese, folate, carrot juice, strawberries, dates, cherries, prunes, liver, lentils, beans, citrus fruits, vegetables, seafood, meat, eggs, raisins.

Flatulence: Pantothenic acid, coriander tea, papaya, peppermint tea, lemon and celery before meals, aloe vera, garlic capsules, pineapple, papaya, dill, digestive enzymes, buttermilk.

Gallbladder Problems: Parsley, wild yams, yellow dock, dandelion, goldenseal tea, carrot juice before meals, horseradish, black radishes, lemon juice, carrots, cucumbers, parsley, chicory, vitamin A, choline, biotin.

Gastric Disorders: Coconut, strawberries, apples, carrots, garlic, papaya, fennel tea, fresh cabbage juice.

Gout: Carrots, celery, cucumber, beet juice, cherries, magnesium, sulphur, comfrey,[8] sage.

Gums: Saltwater, vitamins A, B, and C, potassium, bioflavonoids, raw cabbage and carrot juice, raw spinach juice, brewer's yeast, wheat germ.

Hay Fever: Carrots, beets, cucumber, spinach, celery, parsley, vitamin C.

Headaches: Sage, silicon, vitamin C, vitamin B6, marjoram, chamomile tea, niacin, bayberry, black cohosh, acupuncture.

Hearing: Vitamins A, B, C, and D, raw fruit, green leafy vegetables, turmeric.

Heart Palpitations: Red clover tea, chicory root.

Hypertension: Cut down on sugar and sodium intake and increase raw vegetables. Increase calcium intake and eat more onions, garlic, celery, watermelon. Also, vitamin P, vitamin D, magnesium, choline, vitamin E, selenium, rutin, zinc.

Hypoglycemia: Raw garlic extract, Oregon grape root, licorice root, uva ursi, cayenne pepper, wheatgrass, potassium, kelp, raw fruit.

Immune System Disorders: Propolis, astragalus (a Chinese herb), echinacea root, thyme, rosemary, garlic, cayenne, rose hips, selenium, vitamin E, zinc, bioflavonoids.

Indigestion: Marjoram, chamomile, whey, acidophilus tablets, peppermint, sage.

Infections: Zinc, vitamin A, vitamin C, alfalfa, garlic, onions, echinacea root.

Inflammation (General): Vitamin C, vitamin A, bee pollen, comfrey,[9] aloe vera, chamomile, cucumber.

Insomnia: Magnesium, calcium, pantothenic acid, niacin, zinc, lettuce, potatoes, valerian, hops. (See also *Sleep Disorders.*)

Intestines: Vitamin B, magnesium, yogurt, buttermilk, aloe vera, whey, carrots, spinach, cauliflower, mangos, pears, okra, bananas.

Irritable Bowel Syndrome: Persimmons, sprouts, carrot juice, beet juice, aloe vera, peppermint tea, alfalfa.

Joint Health: Magnesium, vitamin A, vitamin C, bioflavonoids, vitamin B6, manganese, whole grains, nuts, legumes, tropical fruit.

Kidneys: Corn silk tea, pear juice, fennel, cucumber, carrots, beet juice, parsley, aloe vera, cranberry juice, celery, watermelon, apples, asparagus, celery seed, parsley root, blackberries, horsetail, licorice.

Kidney Stones: Vitamin B6, magnesium, parsley tea, walnuts.

Knees, Stiff: Cherries.

Leg Cramps: Magnesium.

Liver Problems: Choline, goldenseal leaf tea, burdock tea, Oregon grape root, rosemary, milk thistle, vitamin A, vitamin C, chlorine, sulphur, iodine, potassium, selenium, lecithin, zucchini, apples, carrots, wheatgrass, aloe vera, dandelion greens, horseradish, black radishes, asparagus.

Low Blood Pressure: Protein deficiency, vitamin C, B vitamins, vitamin E.

Lungs: Garlic, horehound, flaxseed tea, coltsfoot tea, slippery elm, vitamin E, comfrey,[10] thyme, hyssop, kefir, white onions, wintergreen tea before retiring.

Memory Loss: Soybeans, vitamin B, choline, ginseng, fo ti and gotu kola (Chinese herbs).

Menstruation: Silicon, phosphorous, potassium, blueberries, huckleberries, chamomile tea, raspberry leaf tea.

Metabolism: Iodine.

Migraine: Vitamin C, vitamin B, chamomile, yogurt with wheat germ, feverfew tea, lecithin, niacin, aloe vera.

Miscarriage (Prevention): Vitamin E.

Mucus: Radishes, plantain, fenugreek, comfrey,[11] nettle, fresh horseradish with lemon juice, fennel tea, lemon juice, cayenne pepper. Keep milk, cheese, and dairy products to a minimum.

Muscles: Vitamin C, magnesium, potassium, corn, lentils, lettuce, almonds, lima beans.

Nerves: Vitamin B, brewer's yeast, iodine, magnesium, calcium, copper, niacin, inositol, apples, carrots, celery, citrus fruits, nut oils, olive oils, almonds, strawberries, beef, celery, pomegranate, walnuts, dill, red clover tea, chamomile tea, ginseng, hyssop, vervain, lemon balm, spearmint.

Osteoporosis: Increase intake of dairy products. Eat foods high in minerals, such as sea vegetables, raw nuts and seeds, strawberries, blueberries, raspberries, cabbage, horsetail, comfrey,[12] nettle, parsley, alfalfa.

Pancreas: Vitamin B, iron, zinc, raw foods, digestive enzymes.

Phlegm: Apples or carrots.

Pregnancy: Calcium, iodine, vitamin B, vitamin E, raspberry leaf tea.

Prostate: Pumpkin seeds, sunflower seeds, flaxseed, magnesium, corn silk tea, zinc, bee pollen, horsetail.

Psoriasis: Aloe vera, a raw vegetable diet, raw fruits and vegetables, vitamins A, B, and D.

Respiratory Disorders: Yarrow, skullcap, peppermint leaves, thyme, eucalyptus, red raspberry.

Rheumatism: Cherries, celery, kelp.

Sciatica: Garlic, iodine, vitamin B1.

Shoulders (to Prevent Pain): Magnesium, iodine.

Sinusitis: Sage, slippery elm bark, a tablespoon of honeycomb chewed fifteen minutes a day.

Skin Disorders: White oak bark, burdock, comfrey,[13] goldenseal tea, chaparral, potassium, aloe vera, zinc, carrots, beets, turnips, artichokes, broccoli, kale, watermelon, parsley, sweet potatoes, strawberries, dates, apple and carrot juice, cabbage juice.

Sleep Disorders: Passion flower, skullcap, hops, valerian, licorice, peppermint, lady's slipper, chamomile.

Spine (to Strengthen): Calcium, silicon, magnesium, vitamin B12.

Stomach (to Stimulate Stomach Action): Raw spinach, alfalfa sprouts, catnip tea, peppermint tea, spearmint tea.

Stress (to Alleviate and Prevent): Magnesium, vitamin B2, vitamin C, folate, calcium, iron, zinc, vitamin B6, chamomile, hops, valerian root, vervain, passion flower, aloe vera.

Teeth: Goat cheese, Roquefort cheese, brown rice, whole wheat, rhubarb.

Throat Ailments: Poke root, hyssop, sage tea, slippery elm, strawberries, dates, onions, garlic, honey, pineapple, white turnip juice.

Thyroid: Fruit juice, vitamin A, iodine, zinc, kelp, manganese, seaweed.

Tonsils: Carrot juice, spinach.

Toxins (to Remove and Prevent Build-up of): Onions, garlic, carrots, apples, beet tops and beet juice, aloe vera, comfrey,[14] cayenne, ginger.

Tranquility (to Promote): Dates, strawberries, bananas, figs.

Ulcers: Cabbage juice, strawberries, coconut juice, celery, carrots, endive, parsley juice, alfalfa, avocados, vitamin B6, vitamin C, vitamin B, licorice, lima beans, okra.

Urinary Tract Disorders: Uva ursi, red raspberry leaf tea, carrots, cucumber, apples, coconut, cranberries, parsley juice, manganese, corn silk tea, garlic, parsley.

Uterine Disorders: Raspberry leaf tea.

Varicose Veins: Vitamin E, vitamin C, calcium, B vitamins.

Yeast: Cranberries.

Appendix B
How to Use This Book

The CD-ROM that accompanies this book will provide you with a copy of your birth chart along with an interpretation of your chart in regard to health. You should first follow the instructions in Appendix D: Create a Wellness Report Using the CD-ROM. This will allow you to create a copy of your birth chart and the health report that accompanies it. For those of you who do not know your exact time of birth, it is recommended that for the time of birth you enter either 6:00 AM or 12:00 noon.

First you will want to examine a printout of your birth chart to familiarize yourself with the signs of the zodiac and the planetary symbols for the planets. You will also note that you are given the sign and house position of each planet in your chart. This includes the sign rising in your chart, which is the cusp of the first house, or the Ascendant.

Then turn to the report generated by the accompanying CD-ROM, which provides an interpretation of the planets in your chart as to house and sign position, beginning with the Sun and ending with Pluto. The information on your Sun sign will give you clues as to your eating habits, vitality, and personality habits that affect your health. As you read your report, you will learn about the sign your Moon falls in and how your emotions can affect your overall health. Positive emotions can have a positive effect on health. Understanding your emotional attitude based on your natal chart is one more step in achieving better health. As you study the sign the planet Mars was in at your birth, you will learn more about how you could be overworking that part of your body.

A weak point in the body can be represented by the sign placement of Saturn. As you read in your printout about the sign placement of your natal Saturn, you will have a clue as to the parts of the body that need to be nourished, and you can begin to take measures to build them up. Nutritional remedies are mentioned throughout the book and in appendix A.

You can also look for any houses that contain three or more planets in your chart and then refer to chapter 6 to learn about the health disorders associated with the houses in your chart.

In your personal wellness report, you will read about the meaning of your rising sign, which is called the Ascendant. The Ascendant is also referred to as the cusp of the first house in your birth chart. Learning about your rising sign, which represents the physical body, will provide valuable information on ways to improve your health. (It is necessary to have your exact time of birth to get an accurate Ascendant.)

To get more information, you will want to find your planetary aspects, which are the lines drawn in the center of your chart wheel. You can find the symbol for each type of aspect in the lower-left grid. Then turn to chapter 5 to read about your personal aspect combinations. You can also examine your chart for any planets in your first house. Then turn to chapter 6 to read the information on a particular planet in the first house.

You can refer to the sample chart interpretations in appendix C to see how all the information is presented and utilized.

You will find yourself referring again and again to appendix A for ways to nourish the weak areas of your body. Utilizing your personal wellness report and the information presented in this book will enable you to understand more fully the working of your body and your bodily strengths and weaknesses.

Appendix C
Sample Chart Interpretations

The following interpretations for the charts of Oprah Winfrey and George W. Bush are similar to the reports that can be generated using the CD-ROM included with this book.

Report for Oprah Winfrey

Birth Information:

    January 29, 1954

    4:30 AM CST

    Kosciusko, Mississippi

Calculated for time zone 6 hours west

    Latitude: 33N03

    Longitude: 89W35

    Tropical Zodiac, Standard Time

Positions of planets at birth:

    Sun position is 9 deg. 00 min. of Aquarius

    Moon position is 4 deg. 32 min. of Sagittarius

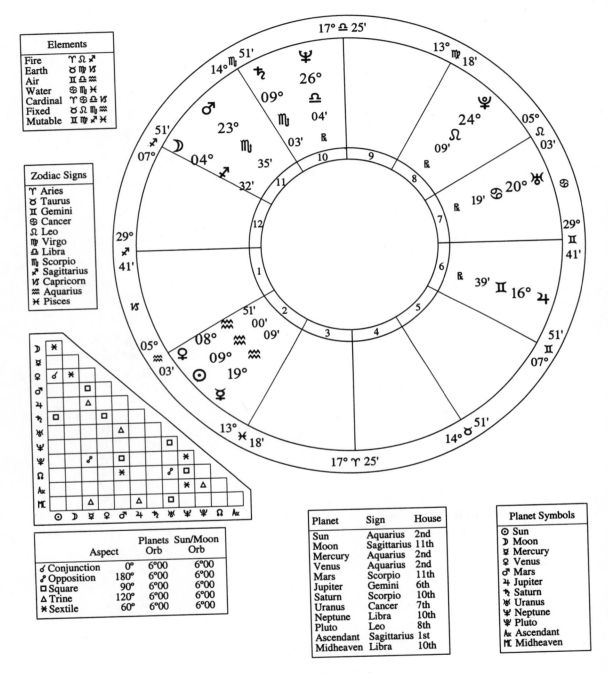

Chart 1: Oprah Winfrey

January 29, 1954 / Kosciusko, Mississippi / 4:30 AM CST

Placidus Houses

Mercury position is 19 deg. 09 min. of Aquarius

Venus position is 8 deg. 51 min. of Aquarius

Mars position is 23 deg. 35 min. of Scorpio

Jupiter position is 16 deg. 39 min. of Gemini

Saturn position is 9 deg. 03 min. of Scorpio

Uranus position is 20 deg. 19 min. of Cancer

Neptune position is 26 deg. 04 min. of Libra

Pluto position is 24 deg. 09 min. of Leo

Ascendant position is 29 deg. 41 min. of Sagittarius

This report interprets the birth chart in terms of health, giving an overall picture of your bodily strengths and weaknesses. You can then utilize your book to get more information on proneness to specific disease states and how to build up and nourish weak areas of the body. As in any type of astrological interpretation, the astrologer looks for a repeating theme before making a final judgment. It should also be noted that the information that follows is taken directly from the book, which sometimes includes references to male and female health disorders.

Disclaimer: The purpose of this report is to provide educational information for the general public concerning herbal remedies that have been used for many centuries. In offering information, the author and publisher assume no responsibility for self-diagnosis based on these studies or traditional uses of herbs in the past. Although you have a constitutional right to diagnose and prescribe herbal therapies for yourself, it is advised that you consult a health-care practitioner to make the most informed decisions. In particular, the herb comfrey is best used externally as an ointment or as tincture drops in water made into a compress. Do not ingest, as some studies suggest that comfrey is carcinogenic in large doses.

The Elements in Oprah's Chart

Low Earth

With a chart low in earth, you can appear to be spacey, dreamy, or unstable. You can be unrealistic or impractical, and you do not manage your time well. Others may see you as unreliable. There is a need to deal with the tangible, practical world.

You can be out of touch with the needs of your body and ignore warning signals of a potential health disorder. You may eat on the run or skip meals. You do not always get enough outdoor exercise or sunlight. You may have poor skin tone. There can be bone weakness, which is helped by exercise and a diet containing sufficient vitamins and minerals. You can be helped by grounding techniques such as a regular schedule of eating, sleeping, and relaxing. Other grounding techniques include gardening or communing more with nature, perhaps by taking a trip to a national park or driving through the countryside. You can increase the earth element by wearing earth colors such as browns and greens, having plants in the house, and spending more time outdoors. A weekly massage can also increase your body awareness.

Eating heavy foods can ground you. These include root vegetables, such as carrots, potatoes, turnips, beets, and squash. You can also benefit by including whole grains, brown rice, nuts, oils, cheese, butter, garlic, onions, and spices such as ginger and curry in your diet. Ginseng, pineapple, and fennel can be helpful in stimulating digestion.

Excess Air

The air element refers to the circulation of the body, the nervous system, respiration, and communication. With an excess of air in the chart, you are highly intelligent but can be detached and impersonal. You tend to ignore the needs of the body, as you are good at rationalizing. You have an overactive mind, which can lead to nervous exhaustion. Your nervous system is highly charged and extremely sensitive. You tend to be nervous, jittery, and anxious. You appear to be energetic but tend to run on nervous energy, without having any real stamina. There is a strong mental component with excess air, with an inability to turn off the mind, leading to insomnia. Teas such as chamomile, skullcap, vervain, and valerian can help calm the nerves. Activities such as yoga or breathing exercises can aid the nervous system. There can be tics and spasms caused by an overload on the nervous system. You need periods of rest and relaxation to allow the nervous system to recharge itself.

You are prone to ailments such as asthma, anemia, flatulence, and muscle spasms and pain. Peppermint tea can help both muscle spasms and digestive disorders. You may be prone to headaches and indigestion. Excess air dries up water, which can lead to thirst and dehydration. You tend toward dryness, causing dry, rough skin, brittle hair and nails, stiff joints, and diseases such as arthritis. You need to increase your intake of fluids, especially water. You benefit from eating whole grains and taking B-complex vitamins and magnesium.

A medical astrologer would note that the combination of low earth and excess air increases lightness and can be helped by grounding techniques such as gardening, cooking for pleasure, and eating more root vegetables. Taking a vacation without your laptop computer, cell phone, and other modern conveniences can help recharge the nervous system.

The Modes in Oprah's Chart

FIXED MODE

With a majority a planets in the fixed signs in the chart, you are reliable, but you can be stubborn and rigid and resistant to change. A lack of flexibility causes you to get stuck in a rut. An overly stiff demeanor can manifest as stiffness in the body. Fixed-type illnesses can be cumulative in nature, resulting in growths, cysts, blockages, or enlargement of a body part. There can be a sluggishness to the body that can be helped by increased physical exercise. You need variety in your diet and plenty of roughage. You would also benefit from body therapies such as rolfing and bioenergetics. Fixed-type diseases are chronic and can last a long time. It can be a disorder you live with much of your life. The parts of the body affected include the throat, reproductive and eliminative organs, heart, and circulatory system. Fixed-cross problems may be related to problems with the colon or thyroid gland. A diet high in liquids, juices, fruits, and vegetables is helpful. Consumption of heavy foods should be restricted.

To alleviate the stagnation that can result in the body from an emphasis of planets in the fixed mode, the medical astrologer would encourage you to eat a variety of foods every day and to engage in some form of daily physical exercise.

The Planets in the Houses and Signs in Oprah's Chart

SUN IN THE SECOND HOUSE

You have a strong hold on life and much physical endurance. You have strength in your upper body and can gain more strength through weightlifting. You are able to rejuvenate yourself through contact with nature.

SUN IN AQUARIUS

You have a strong constitution and the ability to resist disease. You are intellectually oriented and are constantly seeking the unusual. You are restless and utilize a lot of nervous energy. You are subject to nervous disorders and an uneven flow of energy in the body.

You dislike conformity and are happiest when allowed to express your own individual nature. When forced to conform, you can become erratic and high-strung, with sudden mood swings, or you may experience a lack of coordination in the body. Aquarius rules the circulatory system, and you can be prone to such complaints as swollen ankles, high blood pressure, heartburn, leg cramps, blood poisoning, anemia, and heart palpitations. Circulatory complaints can range from varicose veins to phlebitis. Systems such as osteopathy are an aid to circulatory complaints. Onion and garlic are blood purifiers and aid circulation. Vitamin E and calcium are helpful for venous circulatory disorders. Circulatory disorders are worsened by smoking cigarettes.

You are prone to spasmodic troubles such as convulsions, fits, and epilepsy. Adequate intake of minerals, especially calcium and magnesium, is necessary. These also help calm the nerves. A lack of vitamin B6 and magnesium can contribute to spastic conditions, which are also helped by vitamin E. It is important to get regular eye checkups, as you are prone to eyestrain and other disorders of the eyes. There can be locomotor disorders such as a sprained or broken ankle. You are also subject to rare or unusual ailments.

You can be erratic in your eating habits, eating when the mood strikes or following fad diets that can cause a nutritional imbalance. You should try to avoid foods containing a lot of chemicals or heavily processed foods. Aquarius is involved in the oxygenation of the body, and as an air sign, you need to get plenty of fresh air to keep your body tuned. A trip to the mountains can be rejuvenating. Exercises such as walking, bicycling, yoga, and deep breathing are helpful. You also need a good night's sleep to recharge the nervous system.

Herbs such as passion flower can aid relaxation, prickly ash cleanses the bloodstream and is an aid in ankle sprains, rosemary used externally stimulates circulation, and valerian can quiet the nerves and be an aid for insomnia. Foods that have calming properties are recommended. These include strawberries, mangos, and watermelon, proteins such as eggs, milk, and turkey, and chamomile tea.

Moon in the Eleventh House

You are unique and independent. You have a tendency to overreact emotionally, putting a strain on your nervous system. There can be a weakness in the lower legs, leading to swollen ankles or a sprained ankle.

MOON IN SAGITTARIUS

You have vitality, good resistance to disease, and a positive outlook on life. You have a tendency toward exaggeration and overindulgence and a strong need for emotional freedom. You dislike restriction and are happiest when planning for the future. There is a sensitivity in the areas of the lungs, nervous system, and hips and thighs, and there can be diseases of the liver and blood and a tendency toward gout and sciatica. Garlic and iodine are helpful in preventing sciatica. Dandelion is cleansing to both the blood and the liver. There can be locomotor disorders, which limit your freedom of movement. The hips and thighs should be guarded during any sports activity and during the winter when walking on icy sidewalks. You tend toward shallow breathing and can benefit from diaphragmatic exercises, which aid the lungs.

MERCURY IN THE SECOND HOUSE

You have strong values and can be dogmatic in speech. You are sensitive in the throat and neck area and may experience hoarseness or a sore throat when under stress. You have a good sense of taste and smell.

MERCURY IN AQUARIUS

You are unique and independent. You are progressive and willing to try unusual methods of healing. You can be erratic, nervous, and high-strung and subject to hysteria. You benefit from the use of calming herbs such as bergamot and skullcap. You may experience muscle cramping, pain in the calves or legs, fleeting pains throughout your body, and intestinal disorders. Rubbing on essence of cloves is helpful to relieve pain in the body. There can be circulatory disorders and nerve-related ailments. Systems such as osteopathy are an aid to circulatory complaints. Onions and garlic are blood purifiers and aid circulation. Calcium and magnesium are helpful in preventing nerve-related ailments. The combination of Mercury in Aquarius is also associated with speech defects, which can be helped by a speech therapist.

VENUS IN THE SECOND HOUSE

You have a strong sensual nature and a good sense of taste and smell. You have a tendency toward self-indulgence in food and drink. You are prone to disorders in the neck and throat area and have a tendency to choke or gag on food.

Venus in Aquarius

You are prone to disorders of the blood due to poor blood circulation. This can lead to swollen ankles, cold extremities, or blood disorders such as anemia. Onions and garlic are blood purifiers and aid circulation. You are prone to disorders such as varicose veins. Vitamin C, vitamin E, and the B vitamins are important. There can be heart palpitations and an uneven kidney function. Herbs beneficial for the kidneys include corn silk and cleavers that promote kidney action, uva ursi for kidney weakness, and feverfew to strengthen and cleanse the kidneys. Wild cherry helps with nervous palpitations of the heart.

Mars in the Eleventh House

You are outgoing and desire the unusual and unique. You can be high-strung and temperamental and overstrain your nervous system. Pushing yourself too hard and not allowing time for rest and relaxation can lead to a nervous breakdown. You can be prone to circulatory disorders and heart palpitations. You should use care when walking on wet or icy sidewalks, as there is the danger of accidents causing injuries to your lower legs and ankles.

Mars in Scorpio

Remember that the sign placement of Mars is an overworked part of the body, and Scorpio in a woman's chart can also refer to female problems.

This placement can indicate problems with the colon such as a spastic colon, an acid colon, hemorrhoids, and diseases such as pruritus (itching), colitis, and irritable bowel syndrome. Apples, figs, honey, licorice, and prunes all aid the colon. Bee pollen helps prevent hemorrhoids and pruritus. Urinary disorders are common with this placement. Men are prone to inflammation of the prostate, and women are subject to female disorders such as vaginitis, cystitis, and problems with menstrual flow. Raspberry leaf tea is an excellent women's herb. Zinc is essential for prostate health, and the consumption of pumpkin seeds is a good source. Both sexes are subject to diseases such as herpes or gonorrhea, which can be avoided by practicing safe sex. The throat is also a sensitive area, and there can be inflamed tonsils or larynx and throat problems. Herbs such as sage or fenugreek can be used for sore throats, and coltsfoot for hoarseness. You are subject to nosebleeds and should avoid blowing your nose too vigorously.

JUPITER IN THE SIXTH HOUSE

You have good health and a sturdy body, but you also have a tendency to overindulge in food and drink, leading to weight gain. The liver is a sensitive area. You should try to avoid foods containing hydrogenated oils. The lungs as well as the intestinal area can be sensitive. You need plenty of raw foods to promote enzyme action in your body.

JUPITER IN GEMINI

You have a tendency to be nervous and high-strung, with a sensitive nervous system. Yoga and stretching exercises can lower stress. Seawater baths and herbs such as chamomile and skullcap are beneficial. Your cholesterol levels should be watched, as there is the possibility of arterial disease. Supplements such as acidophilus, activated charcoal, and calcium can help lower cholesterol levels. The lungs are sensitive, with the potential for lung congestion, disorders such as bronchitis or pleurisy, or pneumonia. Thyme tea helps eliminate phlegm. You may also experience swelling in the hands and sciatica in the arms. Garlic and iodine are helpful in preventing sciatica.

SATURN IN THE TENTH HOUSE

You are authoritative and disciplined, with much endurance. You are able to follow a strict diet and a healthy exercise regimen, which promotes good health. There is a weakness in the bones and teeth, and you need to schedule regular visits to a dentist, as you are prone to tooth decay. A bone density test when older can give you a clue as to whether there is any bone weakness in your body. You may be subject to aching joints and arthritis in the knees. When it comes to treating a health disorder, you prefer the tried and true and will avoid nontraditional forms of healing.

SATURN IN SCORPIO

Remember that the sign occupied by Saturn is considered a weak point in the body, and with both Mars and Saturn in Scorpio, the Scorpio-ruled parts of the body would be subject to both overactivity and underactivity.

This placement indicates potential weaknesses in the eliminative and reproductive organs. There can be colon stasis, stones in the bladder, retention of urine, bladder problems, sluggish peristalsis, and a tendency toward hemorrhoids or constipation. You can benefit from figs, prunes, licorice, raw spinach salad, strawberries, and apples for eliminative disorders. Pearl barley helps overcome urinary disorders. In males, there can be weakened prostate function, an enlarged prostate, or low sperm count. In females, there can be weakness in the female organs. Pumpkin seeds and supplementation with zinc and magnesium are helpful to the prostate. Bee pollen is also helpful for prostate health. Raspberry leaf tea is a tonic for women. With reflex action to Taurus, the sign opposite Scorpio, you may also find that the throat region is vulnerable, resulting in throat problems, phlegm, hoarseness, and poor thyroid defense. Kelp is an aid to the thyroid, as are foods high in iodine, such as Swiss chard, watercress, broccoli, mushrooms, spinach, red cabbage, and potato skins. Herbs such as sage or fenugreek can be used for sore throats, and coltsfoot for hoarseness.

URANUS IN THE SEVENTH HOUSE
You are individualistic and seek others who have unique temperaments. You have an impulsive nature, which can lead to accidents to the ankles or calves. There can be cramping of the lower legs. You can also experience spasmodic kidney pain and lower back spasms. You would benefit from back exercises to relieve tension.

URANUS IN CANCER
You are prone to a nervous stomach, with an uneven assimilation of food. You tend to have your own daily rhythm and may eat at odd hours, which can further contribute to poor assimilation of vitamins and minerals and contribute to stomach disorders. You are prone to spasmodic conditions of the stomach and stomach cramps and may become nauseous or vomit when under stress. You vary between an overacid and overalkaline stomach. Lettuce, carrots, and celery help promote alkalinity, which is considered conducive to good health. Chamomile tea soothes the stomach, as does cold sage tea. Both ginger and peppermint teas aid nausea.

NEPTUNE IN THE TENTH HOUSE
You are idealistic and can be charismatic and appealing. There can be a weakness in the bones, teeth, and hair, which would benefit from increased minerals in your diet and taking herbs such as silica or horsetail. Toxic substances in the environment can cause a calcium imbalance in your body. You need frequent trips to the dentist, as there is a tendency toward tooth decay. Your knees can be weak, and you may be prone to knee injuries.

NEPTUNE IN LIBRA

This placement can indicate weak or sluggish kidney function or poor filtering of urine from the body, causing anemia and potential problems with the spleen. Toxins caused by a bad reaction to a drug can adversely affect your kidneys, and there is a need for pure food and water. Corn silk tea and pear juice promote kidney action. The electrolyte balance in the body can be off. Eye problems may be due to poor kidney function. Be careful of ingesting too much hard water, as this can adversely affect the kidneys. There can be an acid/alkaline imbalance in the body and a sodium imbalance. Alfalfa helps promote a healthy balance in the body. You should stay closer to an alkaline diet by eating foods such as berries, fresh vegetables, and milk products.

PLUTO IN THE EIGHTH HOUSE

You can be intense and powerful. Your relentless drive can put a strain on your nervous system. The reproductive and eliminative organs are sensitive, and too much stress can lead to disorders such as irritable bowel syndrome or colitis. Women with this placement are subject to miscarriage. Men with this placement may have problems with the prostate.

The Ascendant in Oprah's Chart

Much can be learned about the physical body by examining the rising sign of the natal chart. This is called the Ascendant, as it is the sign rising on the eastern horizon at the moment of birth. In order to accurately interpret your Ascendant, you need to have your exact time of birth. The sign on the Ascendant and the aspects made to the Ascendant by the planets in your chart give much information about the physical body.

SAGITTARIUS ASCENDANT

You have vitality, are able to conduct energy throughout your body, and have good recuperative powers. Your positive outlook on life aids your emotional and physical well-being. You always need something to aim for, as a lack of goals or a stagnant existence causes you to become depressed. You can experience mental and nervous strain from not getting enough rest, which can overtax the nervous system. You tend to indulge in high-fat foods, which puts a strain on the liver, a vulnerable part of your body. The weak parts of your body are from the hips to the knees, with a tendency toward ailments such as sciatica. Garlic and iodine are helpful against sciatica. Older persons should protect themselves, as there can be danger of falls and hip injury. A Sagittarius Ascendant also gives a tendency toward feverish ailments and respiratory disorders such as pneumonia, bronchitis, asthma, and pleurisy.

The Sixth House in Oprah's Chart

GEMINI ON THE CUSP OF THE SIXTH HOUSE

This position gives energy and vitality. There can be a desire to work in occupations that require the use of the mind and are intellectually stimulating, as you can easily become bored. If involved in work you dislike, there can be depression and anxiety. You have the ability to engage in more than one activity at a time. You are good with your hands and need to guard against work-related injuries to the arms and hands. You are also susceptible to airborne pollutants in the workplace, which can lead to respiratory problems such as bronchitis or asthma or allergic reactions. Proper breathing is important for maintenance of health. You are susceptible to lung ailments as well as to fractures of the arms or wrists. Your nervous system is also sensitive, and you are subject to nervous disorders when in a difficult work situation. You do not handle stress well. Mercury rules Gemini, and its position and aspects should be examined.

Report for George W. Bush

Birth Information:

> July 6, 1946
>
> 7:26 AM EST
>
> New Haven, Connecticut

Calculated for time zone 5 hours west

> Latitude: 41N18
>
> Longitude: 72W55
>
> Tropical Zodiac, Daylight Saving Time

Positions of planets at birth:

> Sun position is 13 deg. 47 min. of Cancer
>
> Moon position is 16 deg. 42 min. of Libra
>
> Mercury position is 9 deg. 50 min. of Leo

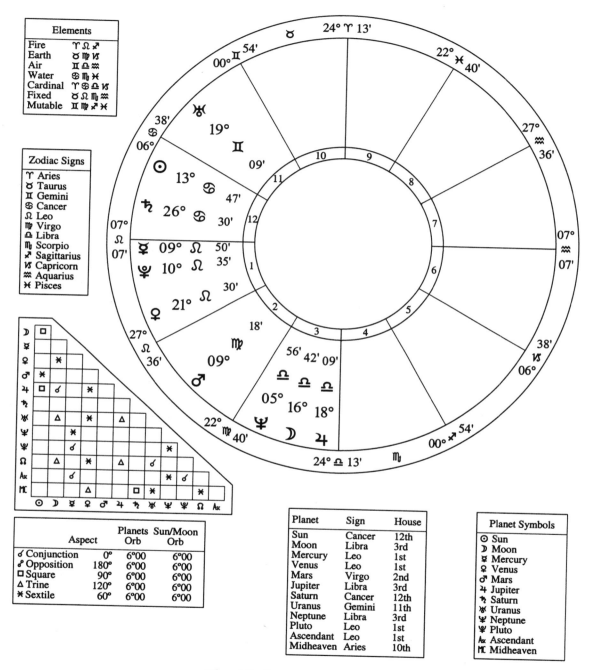

Elements	
Fire	♈ ♌ ♐
Earth	♉ ♍ ♑
Air	♊ ♎ ♒
Water	♋ ♏ ♓
Cardinal	♈ ♋ ♎ ♑
Fixed	♉ ♌ ♏ ♒
Mutable	♊ ♍ ♐ ♓

Zodiac Signs	
♈	Aries
♉	Taurus
♊	Gemini
♋	Cancer
♌	Leo
♍	Virgo
♎	Libra
♏	Scorpio
♐	Sagittarius
♑	Capricorn
♒	Aquarius
♓	Pisces

	Aspect	Planets Orb	Sun/Moon Orb
☌	Conjunction	0°	6°00	6°00
☍	Opposition	180°	6°00	6°00
□	Square	90°	6°00	6°00
△	Trine	120°	6°00	6°00
⚹	Sextile	60°	6°00	6°00

Planet	Sign	House
Sun	Cancer	12th
Moon	Libra	3rd
Mercury	Leo	1st
Venus	Leo	1st
Mars	Virgo	2nd
Jupiter	Libra	3rd
Saturn	Cancer	12th
Uranus	Gemini	11th
Neptune	Libra	3rd
Pluto	Leo	1st
Ascendant	Leo	1st
Midheaven	Aries	10th

Planet Symbols	
☉	Sun
☽	Moon
☿	Mercury
♀	Venus
♂	Mars
♃	Jupiter
♄	Saturn
♅	Uranus
♆	Neptune
♇	Pluto
A⚹	Ascendant
ℳ	Midheaven

Chart 2: George W. Bush

July 6, 1946 / New Haven, Connecticut / 7:26 AM EDT

Placidus Houses

Venus position is 21 deg. 30 min. of Leo

Mars position is 9 deg. 18 min. of Virgo

Jupiter position is 18 deg. 09 min. of Libra

Saturn position is 26 deg. 30 min. of Cancer

Uranus position is 19 deg. 09 min. of Gemini

Neptune position is 5 deg. 56 min. of Libra

Pluto position is 10 deg. 35 min. of Leo

Ascendant position is 17 deg. 07 min. of Leo

This report interprets the birth chart in terms of health, giving an overall picture of your bodily strengths and weaknesses. You can then utilize your book to get more information on proneness to specific disease states and how to build up and nourish weak areas of the body. As in any type of astrological interpretation, the astrologer looks for a repeating theme before making a final judgment. It should also be noted that the information that follows is taken directly from the book, which sometimes includes references to male and female health disorders.

Disclaimer: The purpose of this report is to provide educational information for the general public concerning herbal remedies that have been used for many centuries. In offering information, the author and publisher assume no responsibility for self-diagnosis based on these studies or traditional uses of herbs in the past. Although you have a constitutional right to diagnose and prescribe herbal therapies for yourself, it is advised that you consult a health-care practitioner to make the most informed decisions. In particular, the herb comfrey is best used externally as an ointment or as tincture drops in water made into a compress. Do not ingest, as some studies suggest that comfrey is carcinogenic in large doses.

The Elements in George W. Bush's Chart

LOW EARTH

With a chart low in earth, you can appear to be spacey, dreamy, or unstable. You can be unrealistic or impractical, and you do not manage your time well. Others may see you as unreliable. There is a need to deal with the tangible, practical world.

You can be out of touch with the needs of your body and ignore warning signals of a potential health disorder. You may eat on the run or skip meals. You do not always get enough outdoor exercise or sunlight. You may have poor skin tone. There can be bone weakness, which is helped by exercise and a diet containing sufficient vitamins and minerals. You can be helped by grounding techniques such as a regular schedule of eating, sleeping, and relaxing. Other grounding techniques include gardening or communing more with nature, perhaps by taking a trip to a national park or driving through the countryside. You can increase the earth element by wearing earth colors such as browns and greens, having plants in the house, and spending more time outdoors. A weekly massage can also increase your body awareness.

Eating heavy foods can ground you. These include root vegetables, such as carrots, potatoes, turnips, beets, and squash. You can also benefit by including whole grains, brown rice, nuts, oils, cheese, butter, garlic, onions, and spices such as ginger and curry in your diet. Ginseng, pineapple, and fennel can be helpful in stimulating digestion.

Excess Air

The air element refers to the circulation of the body, the nervous system, respiration, and communication. With an excess of air in the chart, you are highly intelligent but can be detached and impersonal. You tend to ignore the needs of the body, as you are good at rationalizing. You have an overactive mind, which can lead to nervous exhaustion. Your nervous system is highly charged and extremely sensitive. You tend to be nervous, jittery, and anxious. You appear to be energetic but tend to run on nervous energy, without having any real stamina. There is a strong mental component with excess air, with an inability to turn off the mind, leading to insomnia. Teas such as chamomile, skullcap, vervain, and valerian can help calm the nerves. Activities such as yoga or breathing exercises can aid the nervous system. There can be tics and spasms caused by an overload on the nervous system. You need periods of rest and relaxation to allow the nervous system to recharge itself.

You are prone to ailments such as asthma, anemia, flatulence, and muscle spasms and pain. Peppermint tea can help both muscle spasms and digestive disorders. You may be prone to headaches and indigestion. Excess air dries up water, which can lead to thirst and dehydration. You tend toward dryness, causing dry, rough skin, brittle hair and nails, stiff joints, and diseases such as arthritis. You need to increase your intake of fluids, especially water. You benefit from eating whole grains and taking B-complex vitamins and magnesium.

LOW WATER

With a deficiency of water in the chart, you tend to be restless, jittery, anxious, unstable at times, and fearful. You may have difficulty understanding your own emotions, and you can lack empathy. You can have problems showing emotions. Blocked emotions can lead to physical problems in the body that can cause an energy blockage. There can also be water blockages in the body and poor or slow healing.

Hair, bones, and nails can be brittle, and you may have stiff joints and dry skin. You may be thirsty all the time and have to be careful of dehydration. There can be a difficulty in eliminating toxins from the body, which can be helped by drinking plenty of fluids every day. You benefit from drinking fresh spring water.

You need foods that are rich, oily, and moist and can benefit from herbs that absorb moisture, such as Iris moss, slippery elm, and licorice. Diuretic herbs should be used with care. You should eat lots of juicy fruits and vegetables, drink vegetable juices, and include more soup in your diet. Limit your consumption of raw diuretic vegetables, such as carrots, celery, cabbage, and asparagus. Salt is acceptable but not in large quantities.

Having an aquarium, joining a pool club, taking baths instead of showers, using bath oils, going to a sauna, going scuba diving, or swimming all increase the water element. Living near water increases the water element. An interest in the arts can also increase the water element.

A medical astrologer would note that the combination of low earth and excess air indicates a need to build up the muscles to increase stamina, as there can be a tendency to run on nervous energy. This combination also increases lightness, which can be helped by grounding techniques such as gardening and including more root vegetables in the diet. George W. Bush also has low water, which combined with the excess air can make him nervous and restless. The low water combined with the excess air also increases dryness, which can be helped by adding more fluids to the diet.

The Modes in George W. Bush's Chart

CARDINAL MODE

With an emphasis of planets in the cardinal signs in the chart, you can be demanding and willful. You are a troubleshooter, you like to be in on the action, and you have a strong need to succeed. You like to solve problems through direct action. In fact, you propel yourself through life with such energy that you may overwhelm others, causing them to react in a negative manner toward you. People born with a cardinal emphasis in their chart tend to rush headlong into situations, often without thinking, and may try to push themselves beyond the limits of the body. There is a need to learn to recognize your own limits and a need for self-discipline and self-control.

You can benefit from the use of meditation and quiet periods of reflection. Physical disciplines such as yoga and tai chi are also beneficial. An excessive amount of cardinal energy can describe type-A behavior. There is a need to slow down.

The parts of the body that can be affected when you have a majority of planets in cardinal signs include the chest area, stomach, rib cage, head, kidneys, bones, and gallbladder. You may find that some of your health problems are due to a weakness in the kidneys or gallbladder. Illness tends to be acute. When you do have a health problem, you are not afraid to try new treatments or medications. You are also impatient for results.

A medical astrologer would recommend that George W. Bush recognize his limits and find quiet times to reflect and meditate. Cardinal types can handle stress better than fixed and mutable types, but eventually the body can break down from the constant demands made on it.

The Planets in the Houses and Signs in George W. Bush's Chart

SUN IN THE TWELFTH HOUSE

People may not see you as you really are. As a child you might have been shy and withdrawn. One of your greatest wishes is to serve others. You may have an unconscious desire for power and recognition. The twelfth house has rulership over the immune system, which can be a weak point in your body. You may be subject to colds, flus, and viral infections.

SUN IN CANCER

Cancer is a sign of nurturing and fluctuation. It is a water sign, which is considered the weakest of the four elements (fire, earth, air, water), as it is too easily receptive to outside stimuli. However, Cancer has great tenacity and has a strong hold on life. You have the ability to rebound from illness and usually become healthier as you get older. You are happiest when you are able to nurture and protect those you love and can easily become depressed if you do not feel you are giving or receiving enough love.

The Sun in Cancer has to come to terms with its strong emotional nature. Since the changeable and fast-moving Moon rules Cancer, you are subject to frequent mood swings and changing energy patterns. You have a tendency to worry, and, being a water sign, you can absorb negativity from those around you. It is necessary for you to psychically protect yourself from negative vibrations surrounding you, as you can easily absorb not only negativity but also toxins in the air. A healthy diet and positive emotional outlets are aids to good health. You can also mentally surround yourself with an invisible shield that deflects negative energy.

You need to learn how to discriminate between your feelings and the reality of a situation. Your overactive imagination causes you to perceive ailments that you do not have. Misuse of your emotions can lead to moodiness, irritability, and emotional upheaval and can drain your energy. Use your imagination in a positive way to see yourself as a vibrant, healthy individual.

You enjoy good food and large family gatherings at mealtime and tend to overeat. You are prone to weight problems both from overeating and a tendency to retain water, which can be caused by a lack of potassium in the body or an imbalance of sodium. Excess fluid in the body can lead to swollen ankles. You could be helped by vitamin B6, alfalfa tablets, and the cell salt Natrum Muraticum. You would benefit from eating foods such as lima beans, endives, watercress, bananas, and avocados. Eating fish a few times a week is also beneficial. Lowering your intake of juicy fruits such as melons and increasing diuretic foods can help decrease water retention. Diuretic foods and herbs such as broom tea, celery, corn silk tea, grapes, juniper berries, raw onions, and parsley as well as weekly massages can help eliminate fluids in the body and break down fatty tissues.

The Sun in Cancer can indicate a weakness in the breast area, the rib cage, the stomach, and the entire alimentary canal. You tend toward digestive complaints, ailments such as arthritis and rheumatism, ulcers, and anemia. A combination of beet and carrot juice helps guard against anemia. You may experience stomach inflammation when upset, which can be helped by chamomile tea. The sign Cancer is associated with eating disorders that run the gamut from malnutrition to anorexia and bulimia. Having your Sun in Cancer does not mean you will get these eating disorders. Rather, the sign Cancer is part of an astrological signature for eating disorders.

Cancer's natural dislike of exercise can lead to flabbiness. There can be a weakness in the sinus cavities, gallbladder, chest cavity, and pleura of the lungs. You may also overindulge in dairy foods, which can lead to mucus formation in the body. Excess phlegm in the chest can lead to coughing. Thyme is a useful herb for eliminating phlegm and helping the lungs. Following good nutrition and adding two tablespoons a day of raw millet bran to juice or cereal help the gallbladder. Sage and slippery elm bark are aids to sinus disorders.

Women with the Sun in Cancer are prone to female problems such as bloating and swollen or tender breasts during the monthly cycle. These symptoms may be alleviated by cutting down on caffeine-rich foods, supplementing your diet with calcium and magnesium, and massaging with St. John's wort oil.

You are prone to stomach discomfort, which can be helped by papaya tablets, enzyme tablets, and lecithin. You should not eat when worried or anxious, as this can lead to digestive problems. Lettuce is a Cancer plant, which can soothe the stomach. You need to abide by a diet of natural foods and avoid overcooked foods that can ferment in the stomach and cause digestive problems. At each meal, you need to eat raw foods, which contain enzymes that aid your digestion.

As a water sign, you benefit from water therapies. Taking baths, going swimming or sailing, or relaxing by a body of water can recharge you.

Other useful remedies for the sign Cancer include the homeopathic remedy Nux Vom for stomach upsets and nervous indigestion, the herb arrowroot to calm the stomach, bilberry for water retention, cloves for stomach gas, and fenugreek tea to soothe an inflamed stomach.

MOON IN THE THIRD HOUSE

You have much energy and vitality but tend to run on nervous energy. This can cause you to become high-strung and nervous. You love to be busy and need a lot of mental stimulation. You can have difficulty turning off your mind at night, leading to insomnia. You may be prone to mucus formation in the lungs.

MOON IN LIBRA

You have a good constitution, good vitality, and the ability to recuperate from disease. You work well in partnership with others and generally do not like confrontations, which can upset your emotional balance. There can be a weakness in the kidney function, which needs to be built up. There can be an inability to lose weight or edema in the hands and feet caused by weakened kidney action. Corn silk tea and pear juice are helpful to the kidneys. You may also experience lower back pain. Practicing good posture and getting sufficient exercise will help you avoid lower back problems. You are also subject to skin disorders involving swellings and abscesses. Some skin disorders could be caused by a malfunctioning kidney, which causes toxins to remain in the body. There is a need to keep your body in balance through regular exercise, good sleeping habits, and eating a balanced diet.

MERCURY IN THE FIRST HOUSE

You are a good communicator with a strong desire to express yourself. You are talkative and like to write. You come and go a great deal and may experience nervous exhaustion. There can be a tendency to worry, which can lower resistance, or a difficulty in turning off the mind at night, leading to insomnia.

MERCURY IN LEO

You have much exuberance and can be dramatic and forceful in speech and writing. A tendency toward rigidity in thought can strain your body. You also have a tendency toward heart palpitations, fainting, backaches, nervous trembling, and mental fatigue. Basil tea and carrot juice are excellent tonics for the body. It is important to take regular breaks from your work, such as walking or stretching, to avoid strain to the back.

VENUS IN THE FIRST HOUSE

You have good health and a healthy outlook on life. There is emotional balance and harmony. You have some tendency toward self-indulgence, which can lead to the ill effects from eating foods high in sugar that rob the body of nutrients. You are prone to skin problems such as hives when upset and acne from a poor diet.

VENUS IN LEO

You are subject to heart or circulatory disorders. The heart and circulation benefit from lemon juice. There is the potential for heart palpitations, spinal problems, backaches, and hardening of the arteries. A tea made from wild cherry bark or wild cherry syrup can help with nervous palpitations of the heart. Hawthorn is an excellent tonic for the heart. You have a tendency toward excessive consumption of rich and sugary foods, which can upset your sugar metabolism. Your fat intake should also be watched, especially the consumption of fried foods, to avoid hardening of the arteries. Garlic and onions help lower serum cholesterol. Acupressure and massage therapy are helpful in back and spinal problems. Yoga exercises can also strengthen the back.

MARS IN THE SECOND HOUSE

You have good endurance and a strong constitution. There can be a propensity toward dental troubles, especially in the gum area. There can also be polyps in the nose that can obstruct breathing. Be sure to chew your food completely, as you are susceptible to choking on your food. You may also get frequent sore throats and pain in the neck area.

MARS IN VIRGO

You have a tendency toward bowel inflammation, liver ailments, and a hyperfunctioning pancreas. Your overactive pancreas can lead to blood sugar problems. The liver and lungs are subject to infection. Dandelion root makes an excellent stimulant for the liver. Spinach and alfalfa sprouts aid the bowels. Flaxseed tea, thyme, and comfrey aid the lungs. You are prone to disorders such as pancreatitis, gastroenteritis, peritonitis, and appendicitis. The ingestion of raw foods improves the action of the pancreas, helping prevent intestinal disorders and blood sugar problems. There can be flatulence in the abdomen due to poor digestion. Coriander tea is excellent for expelling gas. Dysentery can be a problem when traveling to exotic places, so you should avoid raw salads and peel the skin from fresh fruits before eating. You are prone to accidents in the workplace involving sharp tools, as well as sickness from overwork.

JUPITER IN THE THIRD HOUSE

You are energetic and robust, self-expressive and active. The lungs are a sensitive area, and there can also be a tendency toward tonsillitis. There can be swellings in the hips or thighs. The liver is also a sensitive part of your body.

JUPITER IN LIBRA

You may have a desire for foods high in sugar or fat, leading to problems in fat assimilation or glucose production. There can be weight gain and a tendency toward diabetes. Diabetes can be controlled by sensible eating. It is better to eat numerous small meals rather than three large ones a day, cut down on starchy foods, and increase essential fatty acids in your diet—sesame, sunflower, safflower, or flaxseed oil. There can be unsatisfactory adrenal and kidney activity. Blood impurities can lead to skin disease. A drink made by juicing romaine lettuce with carrots stimulates the adrenals. Red clover tea is a blood purifier. The kidneys are sensitive, and there can be cholesterol deposits in the kidney tubules or fever due to a disorder in the kidneys. Corn silk tea and pear juice promote kidney action.

SATURN IN THE TWELFTH HOUSE

You work well when alone and at times seem to thrive on isolation. Your immune system can be weak and needs to be built up. There can be a weakness in the foot area and conditions such as foot deformity, fallen arches, bunions, cold feet, and accidents causing injury to the feet. You have a tendency toward worry and anxiety, which can lead to depression. There is a need to cultivate a positive attitude.

Saturn in Cancer

This placement can indicate low hydrochloric acid levels in the stomach, causing poor digestive processes and gastric complaints. This combination is sometimes indicative of a lack of appetite and poor nutrition. Saturn in Cancer is part of a signature for anorexia and bulimia. With this placement, vitamins and minerals may not be absorbed adequately in the body. You should avoid drinking citrus juice on an empty stomach, as this can irritate your stomach. Raw dandelion is good for a hyperactive stomach. Catnip tea helps reduce stomach acid. Marjoram and chamomile are good for indigestion. Anemia can be brought on because the intrinsic factor (an enzyme produced in the stomach) is hyperfunctioning. You benefit from eating foods high in vitamin B12, such as beef, liver, eggs, milk, and cheese. Foods high in iron, such as apples, beets, apricots, broccoli, blueberries, raisins, spinach, whole wheat, almonds, dates, and wheat germ, are beneficial.

With Saturn in Cancer, there is a need to build up your digestive functions. There are different measures you can take to stimulate your stomach. Grapefruit juice acts as a stimulus, but it should not be taken on an empty stomach. Drinking cold water before a meal is also a stimulus to the stomach. If you do not have an excess of fire in your chart, you would benefit from increasing your intake of spicy food to help stimulate your stomach. This includes foods containing spices such as ginger or curry. Refrain from eating late at night, as your stomach doesn't have time to empty properly, causing you to wake up feeling bloated and tired.

Women with this placement are prone to breast cysts or fibroid tumors. Kelp can help the breasts. Women may benefit from taking the herb vitex, also called chasteberry. In both sexes, the ribs are a sensitive area and should be protected in sports activity. There can also be a tendency toward arthritis, stiff knee joints, gallstones, or sinusitis. Taking two tablespoons daily of either raw miller's bran or oat bran improves gallbladder action. Cherries, fresh fruit and vegetable juices, parsley, alfalfa, and watercress are all helpful for arthritic complaints and joint pain.

Uranus in the Eleventh House

You have far-reaching goals and enjoy the company of many diverse individuals. You can be nervous and high-strung and need to find ways to relax. There can be accidents to the lower legs, ankles, and calves due to carelessness. You may experience circulatory disorders.

URANUS IN GEMINI

There can be a potential for cramps and spasms in the hands, arms, or shoulders. Arnica ointment is excellent for muscle cramps or spasms, as is eucalyptus oil and a compress of apple cider vinegar. Uranus is involved with the processes of oxygenation, so this placement can indicate an asthmatic tendency. Asthma responds well to acupuncture as well as to fenugreek tea and aloe vera. Eating lentils is also helpful. You are also subject to dry coughs. Wild cherry extract is good for coughs. Slippery elm is excellent for chest complaints. Gemini has general rulership over all the tubes in the body, so you can experience spasmodic constriction of one of the tubes of the body as well as muscular tics and twitches. A lack of vitamin E, magnesium, and vitamin B6 can lead to spastic conditions. The combination of Uranus and Gemini can indicate that you are high-strung, with a potential for nervous disorders. Chamomile tea and clove tea help quiet the nerves.

NEPTUNE IN THE THIRD HOUSE

You are creative and idealistic. You have a weakness in the respiratory system and are prone to respiratory allergies such as hay fever. There are also asthmatic tendencies. You would benefit from breathing exercises to increase lung capacity. You may also be prone to the negative effects of environmental toxins. You should avoid smoking, as the lungs can be weak.

NEPTUNE IN LIBRA

This placement can indicate weak or sluggish kidney function or poor filtering of urine from the body, causing anemia and potential problems with the spleen. Toxins caused by a bad reaction to a drug can adversely affect your kidneys, and there is a need for pure food and water. Corn silk tea and pear juice promote kidney action. The electrolyte balance in the body can be off. Eye problems may be due to poor kidney function. Be careful of ingesting too much hard water, as this can adversely affect the kidneys. There can be an acid/alkaline imbalance in the body and a sodium imbalance. Alfalfa helps promote a healthy balance in the body. You should stay closer to an alkaline diet by eating foods such as berries, fresh vegetables, and milk products.

PLUTO IN THE FIRST HOUSE

You have a powerful personality, with a tendency to push yourself to extremes. Throughout your life, you go through periods of elimination and regeneration. There can be radical changes in appearance and the use of cosmetic surgery to alter your appearance. You like to be physically active and also enjoy transforming your body through bodybuilding. You may be prone to endocrine gland malfunctions. There can be hereditary diseases.

The Ascendant in George W. Bush's Chart

LEO ASCENDANT

You have endurance and vitality and good recuperative powers. You have good powers of resistance, as the vital energies are well distributed in your body. You have a strong sense of pride and dignity, with a craving for attention. You need to feel loved and appreciated to maintain good health. The heart and circulatory system are vulnerable. You are also prone to middle-back ailments, which can be exacerbated by stress. You need to maintain purity of the blood and see to proper elimination to avoid toxins in the blood. You are a creature of habit, with a tendency to get into ruts at times. You have a liking for rich food, which can raise cholesterol levels in the body. It is important that you engage in an exercise regimen, as you benefit from cardiovascular exercise.

The Sixth House in George W. Bush's Chart

CAPRICORN ON THE CUSP OF THE SIXTH HOUSE

This is a placement that gets better with age. You are responsible and disciplined and need work that allows you some measure of authority and control. When ill, you may experience aches and pains, especially in the joints. You are also prone to colds, chills, digestive ailments, falls, and skin ailments. You may experience uneven energy levels, which can be helped by diet and exercise. You can be a strict disciplinarian and are able to follow a special diet when necessary. Capricorn is ruled by Saturn, and its position and aspects should be examined.

Appendix D
Create a Wellness Report
Using the CD-ROM

First you need to install the program. Just remove the CD-ROM from its folder and place it in your computer's CD-ROM drive. The program will begin to install itself.

If it does not start automatically, click on the Start menu and select "Run." In the Run menu dialog box, type in your corresponding CD-ROM drive followed by the file name SETUP.exe. Typically, the CD-ROM is set up as D:\. The install wizard will run and guide you through the rest of the process.

For an alternate method, you can access your CD-ROM drive by clicking on "My Computer" and then the CD-ROM drive (typically D:\). Double-click on the SETUP.exe icon.

When you double-click on the program icon, you will see a screen called "Managing Your Health & Wellness," which is pictured on the following page.

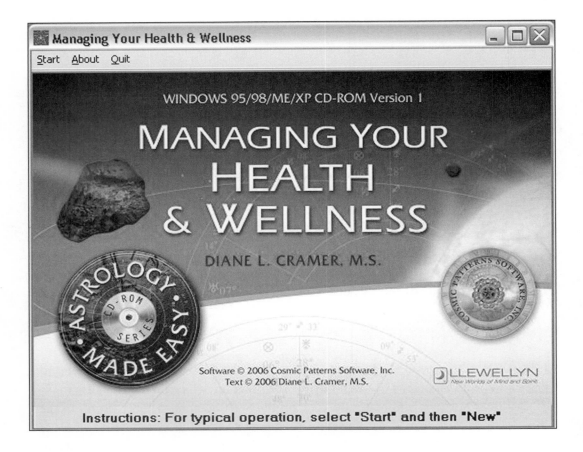

Managing Your Health & Wellness is a basic astrology program, designed around the most sophisticated astrology programming available. Cosmic Patterns, in collaboration with Llewellyn Worldwide, has developed this program to provide you with birth charts (the circle with all the astrological symbols) and basic interpretations of those charts in terms of health and wellness (eight- to ten-page printouts).

Let's discuss the choices you have on this screen:

- The Start menu is used to create a chart.
- The About menu provides information about Llewellyn Worldwide, the publisher of *Managing Your Health & Wellness,* and Cosmic Patterns Software, the designer of the program.
- The Quit menu allows you to exit the program.

Creating an Astrology Chart and Wellness Report

To use your program, click on the Start menu at the top of the screen and select "New List of Charts (New Session)." If you are returning to the program and want to see the last chart you made, select "Continue with Charts of Previous Session."

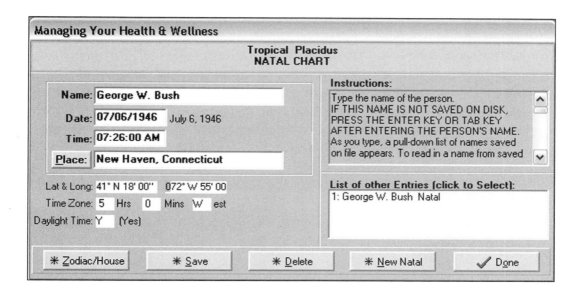

This is where you enter your birth information. There are some simple instructions on the right side of the screen, similar to what follows here. Let's make a birth chart for George W. Bush as an example. He was born on July 6, 1946, at 7:26 AM in New Haven, Connecticut.

- In the Name box, type "George W. Bush," and Enter.
- In the Date box, type "07061946", and Enter. (Always enter the date in mm dd yyyy format.)
- In the Time field, type "072600 AM" (the birth time in hh mm ss format), and Enter.
- In the Place box, type "New Haven, Connecticut" (the birthplace). As soon as you type the word "New," a list will drop down. You can continue typing, or look for New Haven, Connecticut in this list by clicking repeatedly on the down arrow.

You can go back up by clicking on the up arrow. You will see some places you have probably never heard of, but you will come to New Haven, Connecticut. Select it. The drop-down list will disappear, and you will see New Haven, Connecticut in the Place box. You will also see information filled in the boxes below it: the latitude is 41N18 00, the longitude is 072W55 00, the time zone is 5 hours 0 minutes West, and the Daylight Saving Time box is marked "Y."

If your city does not automatically come up in the list, you can use a nearby city from the list. You can also look up your birthplace in an atlas to find the latitude and longitude, time zone, and daylight saving time information, and fill in this information. Generally, a city close to the birthplace is close enough for most purposes and will also be in the same time zone. If the time zone information is different, your chart could be off by an hour one way or the other. Your chart will be slightly different depending on the distance your choice is from your actual birthplace. You can obtain the correct longitude, latitude, and time information from a timetable book for astrology.[1]

The Zodiac/House button allows you to select a different house system. This program automatically selects the tropical zodiac and the Placidus house system. Experiment with the other choices to see what changes on the chart wheel. In this program the interpretation will change only if you select the sidereal zodiac.

Select the "Save" button at the bottom of the screen to save the chart (you can delete it later if you need to), and then click "OK."

Then select the "Done" button. If you forget to save and go directly to the Done button, you will get a prompt asking if you want to save the data. In fact, all the way along prompts appear to help you enter the data.

The report pictured on the next page is what you will see next.

---

1. Here are two possibilities: *The American Atlas*, compiled and programmed by Neil F. Michelsen (San Diego, CA: ACS Publications, 1978); and *The International Atlas*, compiled and programmed by Thomas G. Shanks (San Diego, CA: ACS Publications, 1985).

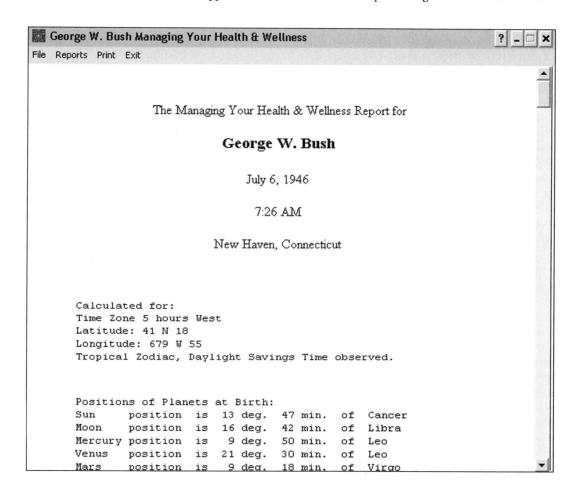

You will see George W. Bush's name and birth data, plus more information lists, and finally the interpretation for the new location you selected. To print this report, click on the Print menu and select "Print."

If you select "Wheel" from the Reports menu, a chart form will appear. In the upper left corner it is labeled "Wheel Style FAC." This form should look just like the one pictured here.

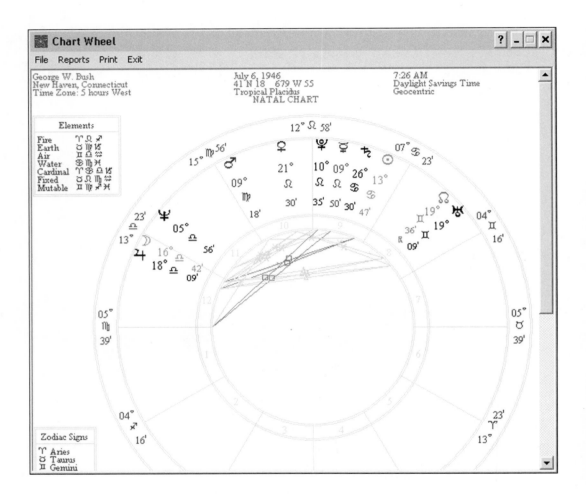

To print the chart, click on the Print menu and select "Print."

To go back to the opening screen, click on the Exit menu and select "Yes: Exit to Opening Screen." From here you can either exit the program by clicking on the Quit menu and selecting "Yes," or you can click on the Start menu to make another chart and interpretation.

Glossary

The following are definitions of the medical and astrological terms used in this book. These definitions were compiled by the author from a variety of sources, including *Dorland's Pocket Medical Dictionary*, *The Merck Manual of Medical Information*, the *Larousse Encyclopedia of Astrology*, and Nicholas de Vore's *Encyclopedia of Astrology*.

acidosis: The accumulation of acid and hydrogen ions or depletion of the alkaline reserve in the blood and body tissues, decreasing the pH.

acid reflux: A backflow of stomach contents upward into the esophagus.

acupressure: A traditional Chinese practice of piercing specific areas of the body along peripheral nerves with fine needles to relieve pain.

adenoids: Pharyngeal (pertaining to the pharynx) tonsil.

adrenal medulla: The central portion of the adrenal glands responsible for production and secretion of adrenaline.

affliction: The condition of a planet that receives difficult aspects from other planets.

Alexander Technique: A technique for positioning and moving the body that is believed to reduce tension.

alimentary: Pertaining to food or nutritive material or to the organs of digestion.

anatomical: Relating to the structure of living organisms.

aneurysm: A sac formed by localized dilatation (stretched beyond normal) of the wall of an artery, a vein, or the heart.

angina: Spasmodic, choking, or suffocating pain.

anorexia: A lack or loss of appetite for food.

aromatherapy: The use of selected fragrant substances in lotions and inhalants in an effort to affect mood and promote health.

arrhythmia: Variation from the normal rhythm of the heartbeat.

arteriolosclerosis: A group of diseases characterized by thickening and loss of elasticity of the arterial walls.

arteries: Vessels that supply the body with oxygenated blood.

Ascendant: The degree of the zodiac rising at the eastern horizon of the birthplace at the moment of birth.

aspect: An angular relationship between two planets or important points on the zodiac; one of a set of specific angles.

astigmatism: A visual defect in which the unequal curvature of one or more refractive surfaces of the eye, usually the cornea, prevents light rays from focusing clearly at one point on the retina, resulting in blurred vision.

Bell's palsy: An abnormality of the facial nerve that leads to sudden weakness or paralysis of the muscles on one side of the face.

bile: A digestive juice produced by the liver and stored in the gallbladder.

bioenergetics: A system of therapy that combines breathing and body exercises, psychological therapy, and the free expression of impulses and emotions and that is held to increase well-being by releasing blocked physical and psychic energy.

biofeedback: The technique of using monitoring devices to furnish information regarding an autonomic bodily function, such as the heart rate or blood pressure, in an attempt to gain some voluntary control over that function. It may be used clinically to treat certain conditions, such as hypertension and migraine headache.

blood poisoning: A systemic disease caused by pathogenic organisms or their toxins in the bloodstream.

bronchi: Plural of *bronchus*—one of the larger passages conveying air to a lung or within the lung.

bulimia: Episodic binge eating usually followed by behavior designed to negate the caloric intake of the ingested food. This can be exhibited by purging methods such as self-induced vomiting or laxative abuse or by excessive exercise or fasting.

bunion: An enlarged prominence on the inner aspect of the first metatarsal, resulting in displacement of the great toe.

bursitis: Inflammation of a *bursa*—a fluid-filled sac or sac-like cavity situated in places in tissues where friction would otherwise occur.

calcification: The deposit of calcium salts in a tissue.

candida: A genus of yeast-like fungi that is commonly part of the normal flora of the mouth, skin, intestinal tract, and vagina but can cause a variety of infections.

candidiasis: Infection by fungi.

capillaries: Minute blood vessels that connect the arteries and veins.

cardinal: One of the three qualities, or modes, that characterize the signs of the zodiac and that are characterized by outgoing energy, self-initiative, and activity. The other two modes are fixed and mutable. Cardinal signs can be hyper and impatient and are associated with a lack of staying power.

cardinal cross: The signs Aries, Libra, Cancer, and Capricorn, which are square and opposite each other in the zodiac.

carpal tunnel syndrome: Numbness, tingling, and pain in the first three fingers and thumb side of the hand that results from compression of the median nerve that travels through the wrist, supplying the thumb side of the hand.

cartilage: A specialized fibrous connective tissue present in adults and forming the temporary skeleton in the embryo, providing a model in which the bones develop.

cataracts: Opacity of the lens or capsule of the eye, causing impairment of vision or blindness.

catarrh: Inflammation of a mucous membrane, particularly of the head and throat, with discharge of mucus.

cecum: The first part of the large intestine.

cell salts: Inorganic substances found in the blood necessary for rebuilding and healing processes in the body.

cholesterol: A crystalline substance of a fatty nature that is found in the brain, nerves, liver, blood, and bile.

cirrhosis: Tissue inflammation of an organ, particularly the liver.

colitis: Inflammation of the colon.

collagen: A component of connective tissue.

conjunctivitis: Inflammation of the transparent membrane that covers the inner surface of the eyelid and the eyeball itself.

cornea: The transparent anterior part of the eye.

coronary artery: Either of two arteries that originate in the aorta and supply blood to the muscular tissue of the heart.

Crohn's disease: Inflammation of a portion of the small intestine and characterized by abdominal pain, ulceration, and fibrous tissue build-up.

cusp: The degree of the ecliptic marking the beginning of a sign of the zodiac and thus dividing that sign from the one that precedes it; the point regarded by most astrologers as the imaginary boundary that marks the beginning of a house in a birth chart and thus distinguishes it from the preceding house.

cyst: A sac containing fluid or semi-solid matter.

cystitis: Inflammation of the urinary bladder.

diabetes mellitus: A chronic syndrome of impaired carbohydrate, protein, and fat metabolism owing to insufficient secretion of insulin. It occurs in two forms, Type 1 and Type II, which differ in etiology, pathology, genetics, age of onset, and treatment.

diaphragm: The muscular membranous partition separating the abdominal and thoracic cavities and serving as a major muscle aiding inhalation.

distillation: The process of vaporizing and condensing a substance to purify it or to separate a volatile substance from less volatile substances.

diuretic: Increasing urine excretion or the amount of urine.

diverticulitis: Inflammation of a *diverticulum*—finger-like projections that protrude from the colon wall.

duodenitis: Inflammation of the duodenum; a common condition often associated with excess excretion of acid in the stomach.

duodenum: The first portion of the small intestine, which begins at the lower end of the stomach.

dysentery: Any of a number of disorders marked by inflammation of the intestines, especially the colon.

dyslexia: Impairment of the ability to read, write, and spell words despite the ability to see and recognize letters.

eczema: A superficial inflammatory process involving primarily the epidermis marked by redness, itching, seeping, oozing, and scaling.

edema: Excess fluid accumulation in the body tissues, manifested by swelling.

electrolytes: Substances capable of conducting electricity in the body, such as acids and salts.

elements: The four fundamental substances—fire, earth, air, and water—which provide one of the two primary classifications of the signs of the zodiac. See *modalities (modes)* for a definition of the other classification.

emphysema: A pathologic accumulation of air in tissues or organs.

endocarditis: Inflammatory alterations of the endocardium.

endocardium: The lining membranes of the cavities of the heart and the connective tissue bed on which the heart lies.

enzymes: Proteins produced by living cells that are capable of inducing chemical changes in other substances; e.g., digestive enzymes.

Eustachian tubes: Either of the paired tubes connecting the middle ears to the nasopharynx; equalize air pressure on the two sides of the eardrum.

Fallopian tubes: Either of a pair of tubes conducting the egg from the ovary to the uterus.

femur: The thigh bone originating in the hip and extending down to the knee.

filtration: Passage through a filter or other material that prevents the entry of certain molecules, particles, or substances.

fistula: An abnormal passage between two internal organs or from an internal organ to the body surface.

fixed: One of the three qualities, or modes, that characterize the signs of the zodiac, the other two being cardinal and mutable. Fixed signs are characterized by persistence, resourcefulness, and magnetism. Negatively, they are associated with rigidity and resistance to change.

fixed cross: The fixed signs Leo, Aquarius, Taurus, and Scorpio, which are square and opposite each other in the zodiac.

gastritis: Inflammation of the stomach.

gastroenteritis: Inflammation of the stomach and intestines.

gland: An aggregation of cells in the body that manufacture secretions.

glaucoma: A group of eye diseases characterized by an increase of intra-ocular pressure, causing pathological changes in the optic disk and typical visual field defects.

glucose: A monosaccharide sugar in the blood that serves as the major energy source of the body; it occurs in most plant and animal tissue; also called blood sugar.

gluten: The protein of wheat and wheat grain that gives dough its tough, elastic character.

goiter: Enlargement of the thyroid gland, causing a swelling in the front part of the neck.

gout: A group of disorders causing acute inflammatory arthritis.

hernia: Protrusion of a portion of an organ or tissue through an abnormal opening.

hiatus hernia: Protrusion of any structure through the esophageal hiatus of the diaphragm.

homeopathy: A system of therapy based on the administration of minute doses of drugs that in healthy persons are capable of producing symptoms like those of the disease treated.

hormone: A substance formed by one organ and conveyed by the blood to stimulate other organs.

hydrochloric acid: A highly corrosive mineral acid that is a constituent of gastric juices.

incontinence: Inability to control excretory functions.

inguinal: Pertaining to the groin.

inguinal hernia: Hernia in the inguinal canal.

intestine: The portion of the digestive tract extending from the stomach to the anus.

intrinsic factor: An enzyme produced in the stomach.

irritable bowel syndrome: Recurrent abdominal pain and diarrhea (often alternating with periods of constipation); often associated with emotional stress.

larynx: The voice box, which is located in the throat.

lumbago: Lower back pain.

lumbar: Pertaining to the loins.

lymph: A transparent, usually slightly yellow, often opalescent liquid found within the lymphatic vessels and collected from tissues from all parts of the body and returned to the blood via the lymphatic system.

lymphatic system: A group of vessels throughout the body that carry white blood cells, which provide a defense against infection.

mastitis: Inflammation of the breast.

metabolism: The series of chemical changes in the body by which life is maintained.

modalities (modes): Also called *modes* or *qualities*; the three types of energy—cardinal, fixed and mutable—which provide one of the two primary classifications of the signs of the zodiac, the other being the elements.

mutable: One of the three qualities, or modes, that characterize the signs of the zodiac, the other two being cardinal and fixed. Mutable signs are characterized by changeability, adaptability, and service. Negatively, they are associated with instability and diffusion.

mutable cross: The signs Gemini, Sagittarius, Virgo, and Pisces, which are square and opposite each other in the zodiac.

myocarditis: Inflammation of the heart muscle.

myocardium: The heart muscle.

nephritic: Pertaining to the kidneys; renal.

neuralgia: Paroxysmal pain extending along the course of one or more nerves.

neuritis: Inflammation of a nerve.

neurological: Having to do with the nervous system.

orb: A spherical space of variable size surrounding a planet or an important point within which an aspect is considered to be potent.

osteomalacia: A disease occurring mostly in adult women that results from a deficiency in vitamin D or calcium and is characterized by a softening of the bones, with accompanying pain and weakness.

osteopathy: A system of therapy based on the theory that the body is capable of making its own remedies against disease and other toxic conditions when it is in normal structural relationship and has favorable environmental conditions and adequate nutrition.

osteoporosis: A disease in which the bones become extremely porous, are subject to fracture, and heal slowly, occurring especially in women following menopause and often leading to curvature of the spine from vertebral collapse.

palpitation: A subjective sensation of an unduly rapid or irregular heartbeat.

pancreas: A gland located behind the stomach and attached to the small intestines that secretes insulin and digestive enzymes.

pancreatitis: Inflammation of the pancreas.

Parkinson's disease: A slowly progressing degenerative disorder of the nervous system; Parkinson's disease has several distinguishing characteristics: tremor (shaking) when at rest, sluggish initiation of movement, and muscle rigidity.

paroxysm: A sudden recurring or intensification of symptoms.

pericarditis: Inflammation of the pericardium.

pericardium: The sac enclosing the heart.

periodontal: Having to do with the tissues investing and supporting the teeth.

peristalsis: The wormlike movement by which the alimentary canal or other tubular organs propel their contents, consisting of a wave of contractions.

peritoneum: The serous membrane lining the walls of the abdominal and pelvic cavities.

peritonitis: Inflammation of the peritoneum, which may be due to chemical irritation or bacterial invasion.

pharyngeal: Pertaining to the pharynx.

pharynx: Upper back portion of the throat.

phlebitis: Inflammation of a vein.

phlegm: Glutinous or sticky mucus excreted in abnormally large quantities from the respiratory tract.

physiology: The science dealing with the study of the functions of tissues or organs.

pituitary gland: An important endocrine gland located at the base of the brain.

pleura: The serous membrane lining the lungs and the walls of the thoracic cavity.

pleurisy: Inflammation of the pleura.

polarity: One of the basic ways in which signs are classified; a sign's polarity is either positive or negative. The fire and air signs belong to the positive polarity, and the earth and water signs belong to the negative polarity.

polyp: A tumor or growth that bleeds easily and is usually benign.

pruritus: Itching.

psoriasis: A chronic hereditary, recurrent dermatosis marked by redness, scales, and papules (elevated lesions of the skin).

pulmonary: Pertaining to the lungs.

pyorrhea: Inflammation of the gums and tooth sockets, often leading to loosening of the teeth.

reflexology: A method of massage that relieves nervous tension through the application of finger pressure, especially to the feet.

renal: Pertaining to the kidney.

retina: Inner eyeball containing the neural elements for transmission and reception of visual stimuli.

rheumatic fever: Inflammation of joints and the heart resulting from a streptococcal infection, usually of the throat.

Rolfing: A system of deep muscle massage intended to serve as both physical and emotional therapy.

rulership: The system whereby each sign of the zodiac is said to be "ruled" by one of the planets or luminaries.

rupture: Tearing or disruption of tissue.

sacral: Pertaining to the sacrum.

sacrum: The posterior wall of the pelvis.

saphenous veins: The large system of veins in the legs and thighs that drain the superficial tissues of the lower limbs.

sciatica: Neuralgia along the course of the sciatic nerve, most often with pain radiating into the buttock and lower limb.

serum: The clear portion of any liquid separated from its more solid elements.

shingles: Herpes zoster; an infection that produces a severely painful skin eruption of fluid-filled blisters.

sinusitis: Inflammation of a sinus.

spleen: A large gland-like organ situated in the upper left part of the abdominal cavity; among its functions is serving as a blood reservoir and producing lymphocyte and plasma cells.

sternum: The elongated flat bone forming the anterior wall of the chest.

stricture: An abnormal narrowing of a passage.

tachycardia: Abnormally rapid heart rate.

thoracic: Pertaining to the chest.

thymus: A small glandular organ at the base of the neck that produces lymphocytes and aids in producing immunity; it atrophies with age.

thyroid: The gland in the neck that controls the rate of metabolism.

toxemia: A condition caused by poisonous products in the blood with resultant illness.

toxin: A poison manufactured by bacteria or other forms of animal life.

trachea: The windpipe.

trench mouth: A painful, noncontagious infection of the gums causing pain, fever, and fatigue.

trigeminal neuralgia: Excruciating episodic pain in the area of the trigeminal nerve.

tubal pregnancy: An ectopic (out-of-place) pregnancy developing in a Fallopian tube.

tumor: A mass of abnormal tissue growth, which can be cancerous or noncancerous.

urea: The chief nitrogenous end product of protein metabolism formed in the liver from amino acids and from ammonia compounds found in urine, blood, and lymph.

ureter: The fibromuscular tube through which urine passes from kidney to bladder.

urethra: The canal that extends from the bladder to the outside for the discharge of urine.

uric acid: An end product of metabolism excreted in the urine.

valvular: Pertaining to or affecting the nature of a valve.

varicose veins: Enlarged, twisted, and poorly functioning superficial veins.

vascular: Pertaining to the blood vessels, either veins or arteries.

vein: Vessels that bring unoxygenated blood back to the heart.

venous: Pertaining to the veins.

Bibliography

Avery, Jeanne. *Astrology and Your Health*. New York: Simon & Schuster, 1991.

Berkow, Robert, M.D., Mark H. Beers, M.D., and Andrew J. Fletcher, M.D., eds. *The Merck Manual of Medical Information*. Whitehouse Station, NJ: Merck Research Laboratories, 1997.

Brau, Jean-Louis, Helen Weaver, and Allan Edmands. *Larousse Encyclopedia of Astrology*. New York and Scarborough, Ontario: New American Library, 1977.

Buchman, Dian Dincin. *Dian Dincin Buchman's Herbal Medicine*. New York: Gramercy Publishing Co., 1979.

Cramer, Diane. *How to Give an Astrological Health Reading*. Tempe, AZ: American Federation of Astrologers, 1996.

Daath, Heinrich. *Medical Astrology*. Mokelumne Hill, CA: Health Research, 1968.

Darling, Harry F. *Essentials of Medical Astrology*. Tempe, AZ: American Federation of Astrologers, 1981.

Davidson, William. *Davidson's Medical Astrology*. New York: Astrological Bureau, 1979.

Davis, Adelle. *Let's Eat Right to Keep Fit*. New York: New American Library, 1970.

de Vore, Nicholas. *Encyclopedia of Astrology.* New York: Philosophical Library, 1947.

Dorland's Pocket Medical Dictionary. Abridged from *Dorland's Illustrated Medical Dictionary.* Philadelphia, PA: W. B. Saunders Co., 2001.

Ebertin, Reinhold. *Astrological Healing: The History and Practice of Astromedicine.* York Beach, ME: Samuel Weiser, 1989.

Geddes, Sheila. *Astrology and Health.* Wellingborough: Aquarian Press, 1984.

Gottlieb, Bill, ed. *New Choices in Natural Healing.* Emmaus, PA: Rodale Press, 1995.

Harmon, J. Merrill. *Complete Astro-Medical Index.* Van Nuys, CA: Astro-Analytics Publications, 1979.

Harrison, Lewis. *Helping Yourself with Natural Healing.* Englewood Cliffs, NJ: Prentice Hall, 1988.

Harvey, Ronald. *Mind & Body in Astrology.* Essex, England: L. N. Fowler & Co., Ltd., 1983.

Heindel, Max, and Augusta Foss Heindel. *Astro-Diagnosis: A Guide to Healing.* Oceanside, CA: The Rosicrucian Fellowship, 1973.

Heinerman, John. *Heinerman's Encyclopedia of Fruits, Vegetables and Herbs.* West Nyack, NY: Parker Publishing Co., 1988.

Hoffmann, David. *The Complete Illustrated Holistic Herbal.* New York: Barnes & Noble Books, 1996.

Jansky, Robert Carl. *Astrology Nutrition & Health.* Rockport, MA: Para Research, 1977.

———. *Essays in Medical Astrology.* Van Nuys, CA: Astro-Analytics Publications, 1980.

Jensen, Dr. Bernard. *Foods That Heal.* New York: Avery Publishing Group, Inc., 1993.

Kares, Kasandra. *Encyclopedia of Natural Remedies.* Van Nuys, CA: Astro-Analytics Publications, 1978.

Keyes, Jonathan. *Guide to Natural Health.* St. Paul, MN: Llewellyn Publications, 2002.

Mann, A. T. *Astrology and the Art of Healing.* London: Unwin Paperbacks, 1989.

Millard, Margaret. *Casenotes of a Medical Astrologer.* New York: Samuel Weiser, 1980.

Mindell, Earl. *Vitamin Bible.* New York: Warner Books, 1979.

Muir, Ada. *Healing Herbs & Health Foods of the Zodiac.* St. Paul, MN: Llewellyn Publications, 1995.

Nauman, Eileen. *The American Book of Nutrition & Medical Astrology.* San Diego, CA: Astro Computing Services, 1982.

Raphael's Medical Astrology. Santa Fe, NM: Sun Books, 1991.

Reilly, Harold J., and Ruth Hagy Brod. *The Edgar Cayce Handbook for Health Through Drugless Therapy.* New York: Macmillan Publishing Co., 1975.

Ridder-Patrick, Jane. *A Handbook of Medical Astrology.* London: Arkana, 1990.

Schwartz, George, M.D. *Food Power.* New York: McGraw-Hill, 1979.

Smith, Samuel. *Atlas of Human Anatomy.* New York: Barnes & Noble, 1961.

Starck, Marcia. *Healing with Astrology.* Freedom, CA: Crossing Press, 1997.

———. *Medical Astrology Healing for the 21st Century.* Santa Fe, NM: Earth Medicine Books, 2002.

Warren-Davis, Dylan. *Astrology and Health: A Beginner's Guide.* London: Hadder & Sloughton, 1998.

Weed, Susun S. *Menopausal Years.* Woodstock, NY: Ash Tree Publishing, 1992.

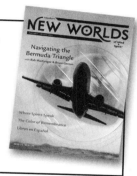

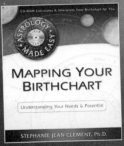
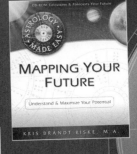
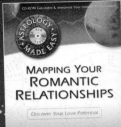
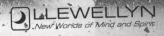

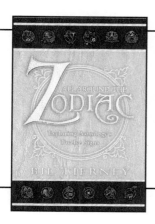

All Around the Zodiac
Exploring Astrology's Twelve Signs

BILL TIERNEY

A fresh, in-depth perspective on the zodiac you thought you knew. This book provides a revealing new look at the astrological signs, from Aries to Pisces. Gain a deeper understanding of how each sign motivates you to grow and evolve in consciousness. How does Aries work with Pisces? What does Gemini share in common with Scorpio? *All Around the Zodiac* is the only book on the market to explore these sign combinations to such a degree.

Not your typical Sun sign guide, this book is broken into three parts. Part 1 defines the signs, part 2 analyzes the expression of sixty-six pairs of signs, and part 3 designates the expression of the planets and houses in the signs.

0-7387-0111-4
528 pp., 6 x 9

$17.95

Astrology
Understanding the Birth Chart

KEVIN BURK

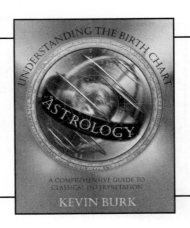

This beginning- to intermediate-level astrology book is based on a course taught to prepare students for the NCGR Level I Astrological Certification exam. It is a unique book for several reasons. First, rather than being an astrological phrase book or "cookbook," it helps students to understand the language of astrology. From the beginning, students are encouraged to focus on the concepts, not the keywords. Second, as soon as you are familiar with the fundamental elements of astrology, the focus shifts to learning how to work with these basics to form a coherent, synthesized interpretation of a birth chart.

In addition, it explains how to work with traditional astrological techniques, most notably the essential dignities. All interpretive factors are brought together in the context of a full interpretation of the charts of Sylvester Stallone, Meryl Streep, Eva Peron, and Woody Allen. This book fits the niche between cookbook astrology books and more technical manuals.

1-56718-088-4

368 pp., 7½ x 9⅛, illus. $17.95

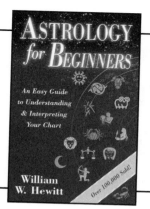

Astrology for Beginners
An Easy Guide to Understanding & Interpreting Your Chart

WILLIAM W. HEWITT

Here is all you need to teach yourself the science and art of astrology! Follow astrologer William Hewitt's easy instructions at your own speed and in your own home as you learn to understand and interpret a natal chart—for fun or ultimately for profit.

Astrology for Beginners will teach you what astrology is and how it works. It discusses signs, planets, houses, and aspects; teaches how to interpret a birth chart; shows "eyeballing" methods for roughly determining a horoscope chart in minutes without using math; explains an easy method to mathematically calculate an accurate horoscope chart; and recommends references to more detailed material for those who want to go further with their studies.

0-87542-307-8
312 pp., 5³⁄₁₆ x 8

$12.95

Spanish edition:
Astrología para principiantes
1-56718-349-2

$12.95

To order, call 1-877-NEW-WRLD
Prices subject to change without notice

Llewellyn's New A to Z Horoscope Maker and Interpreter
A Comprehensive Self-Study Course

LLEWELLYN GEORGE

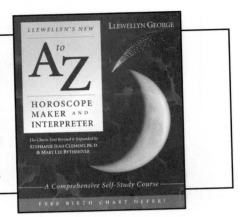

For ninety-three years, astrologers the world over have trusted the *A to Z* as their primary textbook and reference for all major facets of astrology.

Now this famous classic enters the new millennium with a huge makeover and additions totaling more than 31,000 words. Today's generation of astrologers can benefit from Llewellyn George's timeless interpretations, along with new material by contemporary astrologer and author Stephanie Jean Clement. The expansion includes modern developments in astrology as well as a Study Guide, making *Llewellyn's New A to Z* the most comprehensive self-study course available.

0-7387-0322-2
504 pp., 7½ x 9⅛, illus., charts

$19.95

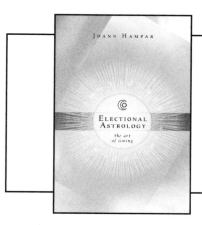

Electional Astrology
The Art of Timing

JOANN HAMPAR

Planning a wedding? Scheduling surgery? Buying a house? How do you choose a date and time that offers the best chance of success? The odds are in your favor when you plan life events using electional astrology—a branch of astrology that helps you align with the power of the universe.

Professional astrologer Joann Hampar teaches the principles of electional astrology—explaining the significance of each planet and how to time events according to their cycles. Readers will learn how to analyze the planetary alignments and compile an electional chart that pinpoints the optimal time to buy a diamond ring, adopt a pet, close a business deal, take a trip, move, file an insurance claim, take an exam, schedule a job interview, and just about anything else!

0-7387-0701-5
216 pp., 6 x 9, charts $14.95

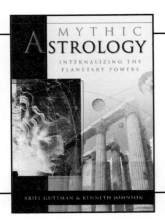

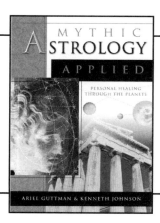

Mythic Astrology Applied
Personal Healing Through the Planets

ARIEL GUTTMAN &
KENNETH JOHNSON

The gods and goddesses of the ancient world are still with us today. They act out in our celebrities, the media, and most of all within our ourselves—often through our dreams and our own horoscopes. Through the planets in your chart you can discover the mythic dimensions of your own life. The authors of *Mythic Astrology* provide a way to do just that in their new book, *Mythic Astrology Applied*. Learn how to contact, work with, and bring harmony to the planetary archetypes within yourself.

This book might have you saying things like: "Now I know why I married a Vesta but really long for a Venus as my partner," or "Now I understand my relationship with my mother; she is a Demeter and I'm a Persephone."

0-7387-0425-3
360 pp., 7 x 10, illus. $24.95

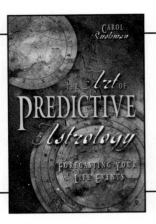